Complications in Orthopaedics
Articular Cartilage Restoration

Edited by
Brian J. Cole, MD, MBA
Professor
Department of Orthopaedic Surgery
and Department of Anatomy and Cell Biology
Section Head
Cartilage Restoration Center at Rush
Rush University Medical Center
Chicago, Illinois

Andreas H. Gomoll, MD
Assistant Professor of Orthopaedic Surgery
Harvard Medical School
Cartilage Repair Center
Brigham and Women's Hospital
Boston, Massachusetts

Series Editor
Henry D. Clarke, MD
Consultant, Department of Orthopedic Surgery
Associate Professor of Orthopedic Surgery, College of Medicine
Mayo Clinic
Phoenix, Arizona

Published by the
American Academy of Orthopaedic Surgeons
6300 North River Road
Rosemont, IL 60018

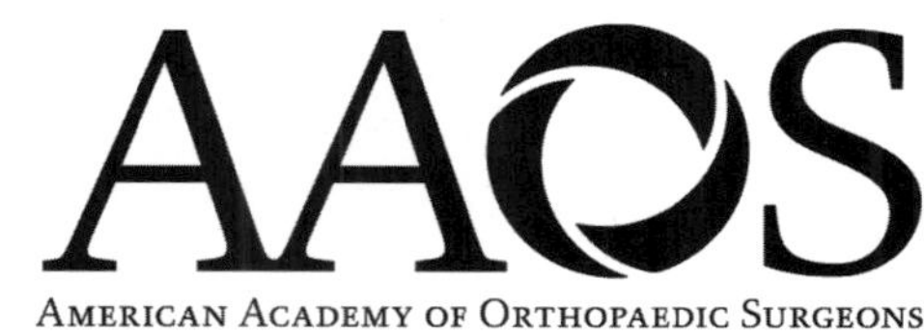

American Academy of Orthopaedic Surgeons Board of Directors, 2011-2012

Daniel J. Berry, MD
President
John R. Tongue, MD
First Vice President
Joshua J. Jacobs, MD
Second Vice President
John J. Callaghan, MD
Past President
Frederick M. Azar, MD
Treasurer
Andrew N. Pollak, MD
Treasurer-elect (ex officio)

Jeffrey Anglen, MD
William J. Best
Kevin P. Black, MD
Wilford K. Gibson, MD
Mininder S. Kocher, MD, MPH
Gregory A. Mencio, MD
Fred C. Redfern, MD
Steven D.K. Ross, MD
Naomi N. Shields, MD
David Teuscher, MD
Daniel W. White, MD, LTC, MC
Karen L. Hackett, FACHE, CAE
(ex officio)

Staff
Mark W. Wieting, *Chief Education Officer*
Marilyn L. Fox, PhD, *Director, Department of Publications*
Laurie Braun, *Managing Editor*
Steven Kellert, *Senior Editor*
Mary Steermann Bishop, *Senior Manager, Production and Archives*
Courtney Astle, *Assistant Production Manager*
Suzanne O'Reilly, *Graphic Designer*
Karen Danca, *Permissions Coordinator*
Abram Fassler, *Production Database Associate*
Charlie Baldwin, *Page Production Assistant*
Hollie Benedik, *Page Production Assistant*
Michelle Bruno, *Publications Assistant*

American Academy of Orthopaedic Surgeons
6300 North River Road
Rosemont, IL 60018
1-800-626-6726

The material presented in the *Complications in Orthopaedics: Articular Cartilage Restoration* has been made available by the American Academy of Orthopaedic Surgeons for educational purposes only. This material is not intended to present the only, or necessarily best, methods or procedures for the medical situations discussed, but rather is intended to represent an approach, view, statement, or opinion of the author(s) or producer(s), which may be helpful to others who face similar situations.

Some drugs or medical devices demonstrated in Academy courses or described in Academy print or electronic publications have not been cleared by the Food and Drug Administration (FDA) or have been cleared for specific uses only. The FDA has stated that it is the responsibility of the physician to determine the FDA clearance status of each drug or device he or she wishes to use in clinical practice.

Furthermore, any statements about commercial products are solely the opinion(s) of the author(s) and do not represent an Academy endorsement or evaluation of these products. These statements may not be used in advertising or for any commercial purpose.

All rights reserved. No part of this publication may be reproduced, stored in a retrieval system, or transmitted, in any form, or by any means, electronic, mechanical, photocopying, recording, or otherwise, without prior written permission from the publisher.

Copyright © 2011 by the
American Academy of Orthopaedic Surgeons

ISBN 978-0-89203-743-8
Printed in the USA

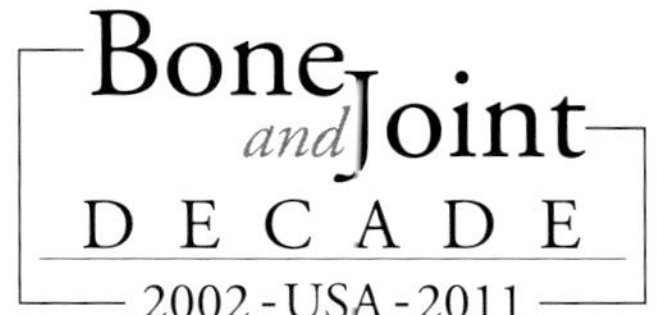

Contributors

Annunziato Amendola, MD
Department of Orthopaedic Surgery
University of Iowa Health Care
Iowa City, Iowa

Joseph U. Barker, MD
Sports Medicine Fellow
Department of Orthopaedic Surgery
Rush University Medical Center
Chicago, Illinois

Davide Edoardo Bonasia, MD
Sports Medicine Fellow
Department of Orthopaedics
University of Iowa Hospitals and Clinics
Iowa City, Iowa

Karen K. Briggs, MPH
Director of Clinical Research
Steadman Hawkins Research Foundation
Vail, Colorado

William Bugbee, MD
Attending Physician
Scripps Clinic
Associate Professor
Department of Orthopaedics
University of California, San Diego
La Jolla, California

Luke S. Choi, MD
Resident Physician
Department of Orthopaedic Surgery
University of Virginia Health Systems
Charlottesville, Virginia

Brian J. Cole, MD, MBA
Professor
Department of Orthopaedic Surgery and Department of Anatomy and Cell Biology
Section Head
Cartilage Restoration Center at Rush
Rush University Medical Center
Chicago, Illinois

Jack Farr II, MD
Medical Director
Cartilage Restoration Center of Indiana
OrthoIndy Knee Care Institute
Indianapolis, Indiana

Nicole A. Friel, MS
Research Fellow
Department of Orthopaedic Surgery
Rush University Medical Center
Chicago, Illinois

Andreas H. Gomoll, MD
Assistant Professor of Orthopaedic Surgery
Harvard Medical School
Cartilage Repair Center
Brigham and Women's Hospital
Boston, Massachusetts

Vasili Karas, MS
Department of Orthopaedics
Rush University Medical Center
Chicago, Illinois

Richard Ma, MD
Resident Physician
Department of Orthopaedic Surgery
University of Virginia Health Systems
Charlottesville, Virginia

Mark D. Miller, MD
S. Ward Casscells Professor of Orthopaedic Surgery and Chief of Sports Medicine Division
Department of Orthopaedic Surgery
University of Virginia Health Systems
Charlottesville, Virginia

Shane J. Nho, MD, MS
Assistant Professor
Department of Orthopaedic Surgery
Rush University Medical Center
Chicago, Illinois

J. Richard Steadman, MD
The Steadman Hawkins Clinic
The Steadman Hawkins Research Foundation
Vail, Colorado

Contents

Preface

Biologic joint reconstruction is one of the most challenging fields within orthopaedics, with rapidly evolving treatment algorithms and new technologies. Reconstruction requires not only mastery of several cartilage repair techniques but also a deep understanding of the indications and techniques for concurrent procedures, such as osteotomies, ligament repair, and meniscal transplantation.

We would like to thank our outstanding faculty for sharing their experience and providing valuable insights on how to reduce the risk of complications, recognize them when they do occur, and address them expediently and appropriately. Even with the best preparation, unfortunately, all surgeons will encounter complications. It is our hope that this monograph will help the reader minimize the impact of these complications and prevent a potentially bad situation from becoming worse.

We also would like to thank our wonderful families for their patience, which we are sure we tested on more than one occasion with this and other projects. Last, but certainly not least, we are grateful for the privilege of working with great people at the American Academy of Orthopaedic Surgeons, who made this book possible.

Brian J. Cole, MD, MBA
Andreas H. Gomoll, MD
Editors

Chapter 1

Microfracture

J. Richard Steadman, MD
Karen K. Briggs, MPH

Introduction

Cartilage lesions of the knee are common and are treated using a variety of surgical procedures including microfracture, débridement, autologous chondrocyte implantation (ACI), and osteochondral plugs. Although many treatment options exist, microfracture has gained popularity because of its numerous advantages including the minimally invasive nature of the procedure, the high rate of success reported, and the relatively low cost.[1-4]

Case Presentation

History

A 56-year-old man injured his knee while skiing. Instability developed in the knee, and the physical examination findings were consistent with an anterior cruciate ligament tear. MRI also demonstrated a medial femoral condyle chondral defect and a medial meniscal tear. Following a preoperative rehabilitation program to improve range of motion, the patient underwent knee arthroscopy (**Figure 1**). The periphery of the lesion was carefully evaluated for any unstable, detached, or undermined articular cartilage. The periphery was débrided back to a stable surrounding rim of normal articular cartilage. The calcified cartilage layer was removed from the entire lesion using a combination of a curet and an arthroscopic shaver, taking great care not to violate the underlying bed of subchondral bone. An arthroscopic pick was used to create evenly spaced microfracture holes at the base of the lesion. The

Dr. Steadman or an immediate family member serves as a board member, owner, officer, or committee member of Vail Surgery Center; has received royalties from Linvatec and Össur; serves as a paid consultant to or is an employee of Össur and Regen Biologics; has received research or institutional support from Arthrex, Össur, Smith & Nephew, and Siemens; and owns stock or stock options in Regeneration Technologies and Regen Biologics. Dr. Briggs or an immediate family member has received research or institutional support from Smith & Nephew, Össur, Genzyme, Arthrex, and Siemens.

© 2011 American Academy of Orthopaedic Surgeons

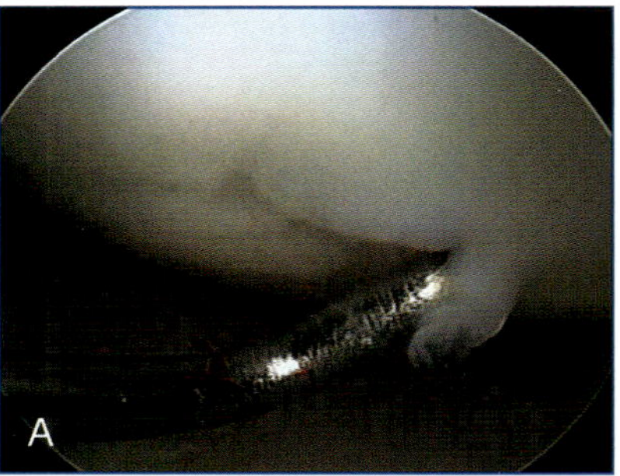

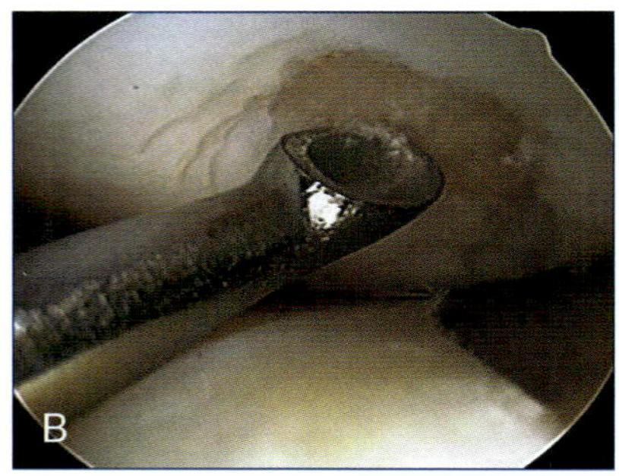

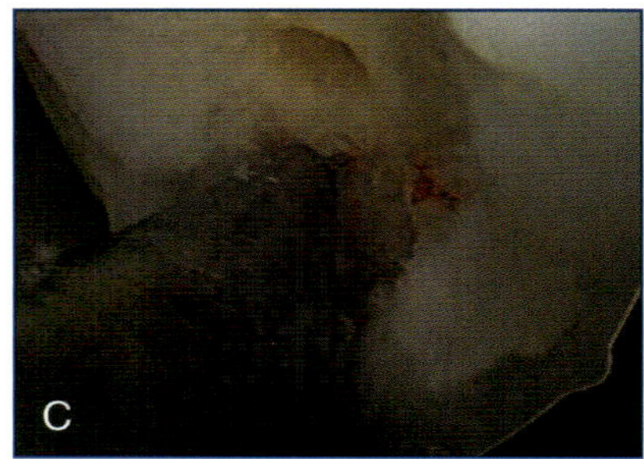

Figure 1 Arthroscopic images of a 56-year-old man undergoing medial femoral condyle microfracture. **A,** The cartilage lesion is probed for unstable, detached, or undermined articular cartilage. **B,** The lesion is prepared with a curet to remove all calcified cartilage. **C,** Evenly spaced microfracture holes are created.

patient also underwent anterior cruciate ligament reconstruction using a bone–patellar tendon–bone allograft and partial medial meniscectomy. The patient returned for follow-up at 1, 3, 6, and 8 weeks; he reported improvement and had progressed his physical therapy. At 8-week follow-up, the patient reported performing deep squats and biking. He was returned to spinning on a bike and was told not to do deep squats until he was completely asymptomatic.

Current Problem

Six months after microfracture, the patient returned following a biking accident. He reported stiffness and recurrent effusion. MRI that was obtained showed subchondral cortical irregularities at the site of the previous microfracture. These subchondral irregularities may have resulted from the bony trauma caused by the microfracture procedure. In addition, the MRI showed scarring of the anterior interval, posterolateral corner, and popliteus.

Treatment

The patient then underwent revision arthroscopy (**Figure 2**). An area of previous microfracture exhibited some coverage with repair cartilage. In addition, a portion of this region measuring 5 × 12 mm was disrupted, with unstable cartilage. This area was prepared and microfractured again.

Outcome

The patient completed the rehabilitation program and was able to return to activity without symptoms.

Discussion

Recognizing the Problem

Complications following microfracture are seldom observed and are for the most part nonthreatening; however, side effects such as arthralgia, effusion, crepitus, and tenderness have been observed and are sometimes recurrent. Overloading is one possible cause of these symptoms and potentially can be corrected by slowing down the rehabilitation intensity.[5] Reoperation is an option if these symptoms persist. Serious complications such as thrombosis are even more atypical. In a study comparing two different postoperative treatments, Marder et al[6] reported deep vein thrombosis of the calf in one patient out of 50 after each group underwent an identical microfracture procedure.

Other minor complications have been documented in the literature. Generally, these complications are related more closely to symptoms experienced following débridement and lavage.[7] If a steep perpendicular rim is made in the trochlear groove during the preparation of the cartilage defect, catching or locking may occur as the patellar apex rides over the lesion. Also, some patients may present with mild transient pain in the patellofemoral joint following microfracture. Patients also may report a "gritty" sensation as they begin bearing weight on the operated knee. Generally, most symptoms dissipate within 3 months after surgery.[1] Another symptom that patients may experience is effusion, which may occur within 6 to 8 weeks after microfracture. This type of effusion is not usually painful and resolves within a few weeks of onset.[8]

© 2011 American Academy of Orthopaedic Surgeons

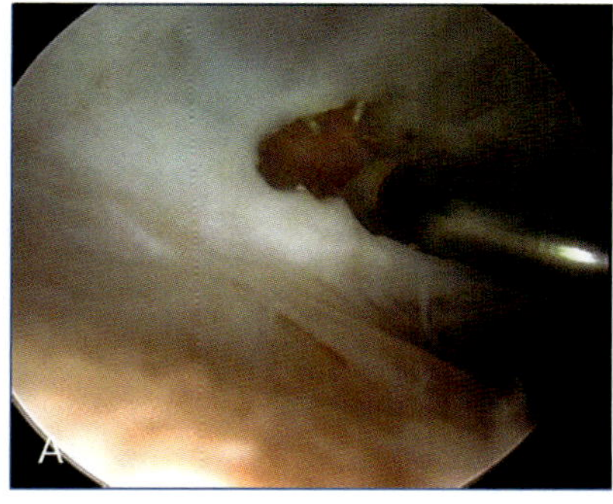

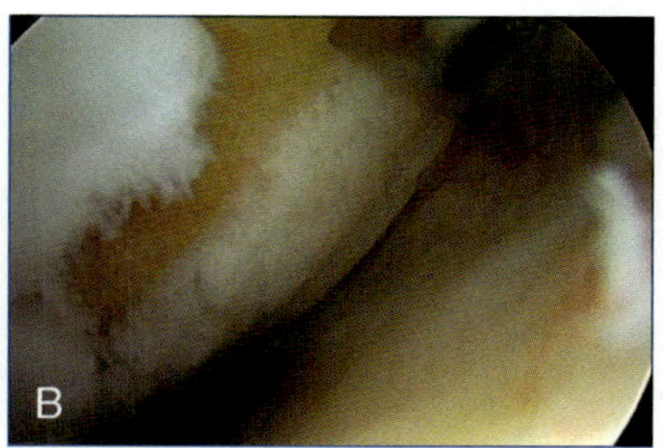

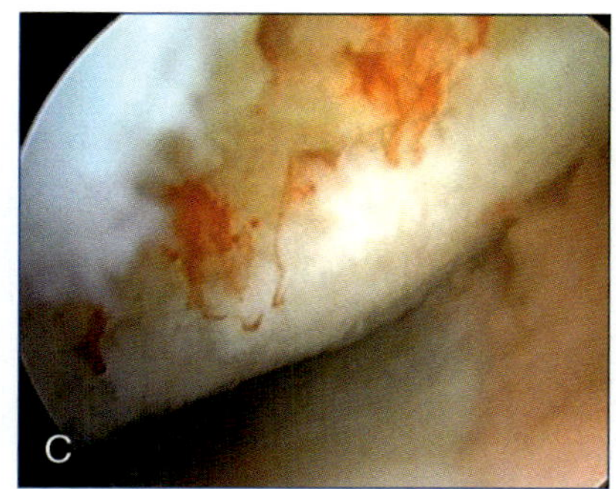

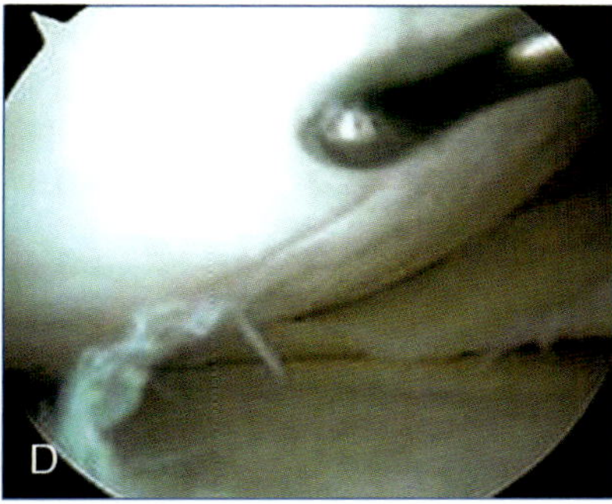

Figure 2 Arthroscopic images of same patient in Figure 1. (**A**) Extensive scarring of the anterior interval is seen. Such scarring has been shown to change the mechanics of the patellofemoral and tibiofemoral compartments. **B,** Medial femoral condyle with no coverage following previous microfracture. **C,** Area of revision microfracture shows excellent bleeding from microfracture holes. **D,** Image obtained 6 months following the revision microfracture shows repair cartilage covering defect. The patient had a subsequent injury and underwent arthroscopy.

Steadman et al[2] studied 75 knees that underwent an arthroscopic microfracture procedure for traumatic cartilage defects. Patients were evaluated annually after surgery for a mean follow-up of 11.3 years. Patients showed significant improvement in Lysholm scores and improvement in Tegner activity levels. No complications were observed in this cohort of patients. The authors attributed the excellent outcomes and lack of complications for each patient to appropriate surgical technique and the use of a specific rehabilitation protocol. Two knees (3%) required further surgery.[2]

Miller et al[3] studied 81 patients who underwent microfracture in degenerative knees and found improved outcomes with no complications. Repeat microfracture or total knee arthroplasty was required within 1 to 3 years after the primary procedure in 5 patients (6%).

Mithoefer et al[5] followed 48 microfractured knees for a mean of 3.4 years. Subjective and MRI data were collected. Repair cartilage fill was good in 13 of 24 patients (54%) who underwent MRI; however, most of the repair cartilage was depressed compared with the surrounding hyaline cartilage. Mild subchondral edema also was noted in 71% of patients. In addition, osseous overgrowth in the form of an internal osteophyte emanating from the subchondral bone was noted in 6 of the 24 patients (25%) after reviewing MRI; however, four of these six patients still demonstrated a good fill grade[5] (**Figure 3**). Although subchondral edema and osseous overgrowth were present in some patients, good to excellent outcomes following microfracture were observed in 32 of the 48 patients (67%).[5] Subchondral edema may result from the bony trauma caused by the microfracture procedure and the slow remodeling in this area. The osseous overgrowth may be due to overly aggressive preparation of the base of the defect, which results in loss of the subchondral plate integrity followed by a bony proliferative response. We have not observed these complications in our patients. Ramappa et al[9] used MRI to study 19 patients with 22 traumatic full-thickness chondral defects and noted incomplete filling of one defect. No osseous overgrowth or subchondral edema was seen.

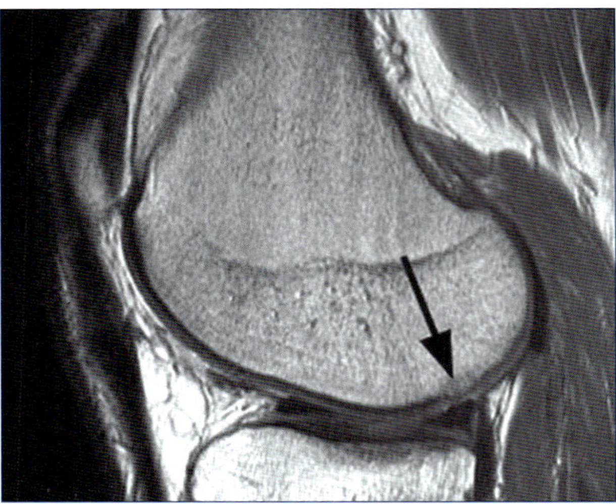

Figure 3 Sagittal fast spin-echo MRI demonstrates marked subchondral overgrowth (arrow) with resultant thinning of the overlying repair cartilage. (Reproduced with permission from Mithoefer K, Williams RJ III, Warren RF, et al: Chondral resurfacing of articular cartilage defects in the knee with the microfracture technique: Surgical technique. *J Bone Joint Surg Am* 2006;88[2 suppl 1]:294-304.)

Bae et al[10] conducted a study to examine 44 patients (47 knees) with moderate osteoarthritic changes in the knee. All patients underwent microfracture and subsequently underwent second-look arthroscopy approximately 1 year after the index microfracture. At second-look arthroscopy, a grayish-white cartilaginous tissue was observed in all cases. No complications were reported, and no revision surgical procedures were required.[10]

Another complication is the need for repeat arthroscopy or revision surgery. Knutsen et al[11] compared 40 patients treated with ACI with 40 patients treated with the microfracture procedure for isolated chondral lesions of the knee; two failures occurred in the ACI group and one failure occurred in the microfracture group at 2-year follow-up. Ten patients in the ACI group required further débridement, and four in the microfracture group underwent débridement. One patient in the microfracture group underwent manipulation and lysis of adhesions due to arthrofibrosis. No serious complications were recorded for this series.[11] At 5-year follow-up, no complications were reported in the microfracture group, and one revision to total knee arthroplasty was reported in each group; the other failures were treated with repeat cartilage repair procedures.[4]

Managing the Problem

Microfracture has been indicated for acute cartilage defects, but the procedure also may be an option for patients with chronic or degenerative lesions. General indications for microfracture include full-thickness defects, unstable cartilage that overlies the subchondral bone, and partial-thickness lesions in which cartilage simply scrapes off the bone when it is probed. Other factors should be taken into consideration when determining patient selection, such as proper alignment of the knee, age, activity level, and compliance with the rehabilitation protocol. Although patient age is not an absolute contraindication, studies have shown that patients younger than 35 years have more improvement than older patients; however, older patients still exhibit measureable improvement.[1-4,12]

Contraindications include axial malalignment without correction, unwillingness or inability to follow the rehabilitation program, inability to use the opposite leg for touch-down weight bearing, and partial-thickness defects that do not fall within the previously mentioned guidelines. Other specific contraindications for degenerative lesions include any systemic immune-mediated disease, disease-induced arthritis, or cartilage disease. Also, patients older than 65 years are contraindicated for surgery because of the difficulty they tend to have with crutch use and the rigorous rehabilitation program. Other factors that may affect outcomes following microfracture include global degenerative osteoarthritis or cartilage surrounding the lesion that is too thin to establish a perpendicular rim.[1,2] A high body mass index also has been implicated as a contraindication for microfracture. Mithoefer et al[5] concluded that a body mass index greater than 30 kg/m^2 will have a detrimental effect on marrow-stimulating techniques such as microfracture.

When comparing microfracture with other cartilage repair techniques, the advantages of microfracture seem very attractive. A well-executed and systematic surgical approach that pays special attention to subtle details, combined with a specific rehabilitation proto-

© 2011 *American Academy of Orthopaedic Surgeons*

col, is pertinent to the success of microfracture and the avoidance of complications. Although the advantages of microfracture supersede its disadvantages, some complications still exist.[5,6]

Preventing the Problem

In the case study presented, the patient did not follow the strict rehabilitation guidelines. The patient resumed squatting activities and biking with resistance before it was recommended. This rehabilitation protocol violation could have resulted in damage to the clot formation or put extra pressure on the healing defect.

Rehabilitation is key to the optimization of surgical outcomes. A specific rehabilitation protocol that promotes the most favorable physical environment for the differentiation of the mesenchymal stem cells has been designed for patients following microfracture. The postoperative rehabilitation program also takes into consideration the size and location of the defect to create a customized rehabilitation program. When other procedures are performed concomitantly, rehabilitation is tailored to those circumstances. Patients also are counseled that they may not experience improvement in their knees for at least 6 months following microfracture. Generally, improvement occurs slowly and steadily for at least 2 years after microfracture.[1] Initially, rehabilitation focuses on regaining motion following surgery. One study showed that patients who used a continuous passive motion (CPM) machine after microfracture had significantly greater improvement in the classification grade of the chondral lesion at second-look arthroscopy.[13] Patients are encouraged to regain full passive range of motion as soon as possible.

Rehabilitation begins in the recovery room, with the patient using a CPM machine as soon as he or she is able. Typically, the initial range of motion is 30° to 70°. This range of motion can be increased as tolerated by the patient. Night use of the CPM machine also is encouraged. The goal is to have the patient using the CPM machine for 6 to 8 of every 24 hours. Cold therapy also is implemented to help control inflammation and pain. Crutch-assisted touch-down weight-bearing ambulation also is prescribed for about 6 to 8 weeks. Patients with smaller lesions are sometimes able to bear weight sooner. Range of motion of the knee, patella, and patellar tendon also is emphasized as an integral part of the rehabilitation program. At about 1 to 2 weeks after microfracture, strength training commences, including knee bends (putting most of the weight on the uninjured leg), stationary biking, and deep-water therapy. At about 8 to 16 weeks, stationary biking is the main exercise. At this point, patients are encouraged to begin knee flexion exercises as well. Patients also are prescribed use of an elastic resistance cord at postoperative week 12.[1,2,8]

Avoidance of complications is particularly reliant upon surgical technique. When performing the microfracture procedure, all unstable cartilage surrounding the exposed bone should be débrided back to a stable rim. A stable rim is indicated by a consistent perpendicular edge of healthy, viable cartilage around the defect. This prepared lesion provides a pool to hold the marrow clot.[1,2,8] Another integral factor for good outcomes is complete removal of the calcified cartilage layer, which usually remains as a cap on the lesion. Thorough and complete removal of the calcified cartilage layer is extremely important, based on previous animal studies. Maintaining the integrity of the subchondral plate is critical, however, so one must not débride too deeply.[1,2,8] As noted above, loss of integrity of the subchondral plate may result in internal osteophyte formation.

Summary

Overall, microfracture has an extremely low complication rate.[2,4,7,9-16] Studies have reported few complications, mostly postoperative pain and swelling, which usually resolve spontaneously within a few months after microfracture.[1] Although other major complications such as deep vein thrombosis and osseous overgrowth have been reported, they are infrequently encountered. When special care is taken to follow the specific surgical technique that has been established, outcomes are typically good to excellent.[2,4,8-11] The calcified cartilage layer and subchondral plate are major factors in a successful outcome following microfracture. A specific rehabilitation program and patient compliance also are crucial for optimum results. When all of these factors are taken into account, microfracture is an effective procedure for primary cartilage repair, producing good results with minimal complications.

© 2011 American Academy of Orthopaedic Surgeons

References

1. Steadman JR: Microfracture, in Feagin JA, Steadman JR, eds: *The Crucial Principles in Care of the Knee*. Philadelphia, PA, Lippincott Williams & Wilkins, 2008, pp 129-152.
2. Steadman JR, Briggs KK, Rodrigo JJ, Kocher MS, Gill TJ, Rodkey WG: Outcomes of microfracture for traumatic chondral defects of the knee: Average 11-year follow-up. *Arthroscopy* 2003;19(5):477-484.
3. Miller BS, Steadman JR, Briggs KK, Rodrigo JJ, Rodkey WG: Patient satisfaction and outcome after microfracture of the degenerative knee. *J Knee Surg* 2004;17(1):13-17.
4. Knutsen G, Drogset JO, Engebretsen L, et al: A randomized trial comparing autologous chondrocyte implantation with microfracture: Findings at five years. *J Bone Joint Surg Am* 2007;89(10):2105-2112.
5. Mithoefer K, Williams RJ III, Warren RF, et al: The microfracture technique for the treatment of articular cartilage lesions in the knee: A prospective cohort study. *J Bone Joint Surg Am* 2005;87(9):1911-1920.
6. Marder RA, Hopkins GH Jr, Timmerman LA: Arthroscopic microfracture of chondral defects of the knee: A comparison of two postoperative treatments. *Arthroscopy* 2005;21(2):152-158.
7. Freedman JB, Coleman SH, Olenac C, Cole BJ: The biology of articular cartilage injury and the microfracture technique for the treatment of articular cartilage lesions. *Semin Arthroplasty* 2002;13(3):202-209.
8. Steadman JR, Rodkey WG, Rodrigo JJ: Microfracture: Surgical technique and rehabilitation to treat chondral defects. *Clin Orthop Relat Res* 2001;391(Suppl): S362-S369.
9. Ramappa AJ, Gill TJ, Bradford CH, Ho CP, Steadman JR: Magnetic resonance imaging to assess knee cartilage repair tissue after microfracture of chondral defects. *J Knee Surg* 2007;20(3):228-234.
10. Bae DK, Yoon KH, Song SJ: Cartilage healing after microfracture in osteoarthritic knees. *Arthroscopy* 2006;22(4):367-374.
11. Knutsen G, Engebretsen L, Ludvigsen TC, et al: Autologous chondrocyte implantation compared with microfracture in the knee: A randomized trial. *J Bone Joint Surg Am* 2004;86(3):455-464.
12. Gobbi A, Nunag P, Malinowski K: Treatment of full thickness chondral lesions of the knee with microfracture in a group of athletes. *Knee Surg Sports Traumatol Arthrosc* 2005;13(3):213-221.
13. Rodrigo JJ, Steadman JR, Silliman JF, Fulstone HA: Improvement of full-thickness chondral defect healing in the human knee after debridement and microfracture using continuous passive motion. *Am J Knee Surg* 1994;7:109-116.
14. Kon E, Gobbi A, Filardo G, Delcogliano M, Zaffagnini S, Marcacci M: Arthroscopic second-generation autologous chondrocyte implantation compared with microfracture for chondral lesions of the knee: Prospective nonrandomized study at 5 years. *Am J Sports Med* 2009;37(1):33-41.
15. Mithoefer K, McAdams T, Williams RJ, Kreuz PC, Mandelbaum BR: Clinical efficacy of the microfracture technique for articular cartilage repair in the knee: An evidence-based systematic analysis. *Am J Sports Med* 2009;37(10):2053-2063.
16. Mithoefer K, Williams RJ III, Warren RF, Wickiewicz TL, Marx RG: High-impact athletics after knee articular cartilage repair: A prospective evaluation of the microfracture technique. *Am J Sports Med* 2006;34(9):1413-1418.

© 2011 American Academy of Orthopaedic Surgeons

Chapter 2

Osteochondral Autograft Transplantation

Luke S. Choi, MD
Richard Ma, MD
Mark D. Miller, MD

Introduction

The treatment of osteochondral injuries of the knee continues to challenge orthopaedic surgeons. One option for treatment is OAT, which involves the transfer of plugs of intact cartilage and subchondral bone from an area of low load-bearing to a full-thickness lesion in another area of the knee. The procedure has gained popularity because of its low cost, durable repair tissue, single-stage technique, and good results in outcome studies. Second-look arthroscopy has shown good healing at the graft site, smooth gliding surfaces, and histologic evidence of hyaline cartilage and viable chondrocytes. OAT has provided good results in young athletes and compares favorably with other treatments for osteochondral lesions. When performed correctly and in the right patient, OAT provides an excellent option for the treatment of full-thickness osteochondral defects with durable and predictable results with respect to pain relief and return to activity. Donor-site morbidity is the most frequently reported complication, although its occurrence is rare in most follow-up studies. Although donor tissue is readily accessible, the limited amount available for harvest restricts the defect size that can be addressed to 1 to 4 cm^2. The most proximal medial and lateral aspects of the femoral trochlea are the main donor sites for this procedure.

OAT is an effective method for treating patients with symptomatic full-thickness chondral defects of the femoral condyles. It has several advantages. First, because the hyaline cartilage is harvested in the form of osteochondral grafts during the index procedure, the technique does not depend on chondrocyte proliferation, matrix implantation, or mesenchymal cell differentiation for the restoration of articular cartilage. The method is not laboratory dependent,

---

Dr. Miller or an immediate family member serves as a board member, owner, officer, or committee member of Miller Orthopaedic Research and Education (a nonprofit organization). Neither of the following authors nor any immediate family member has received anything of value from or owns stock in a commercial company or institution related directly or indirectly to the subject of this chapter: Dr. Choi and Dr. Ma.

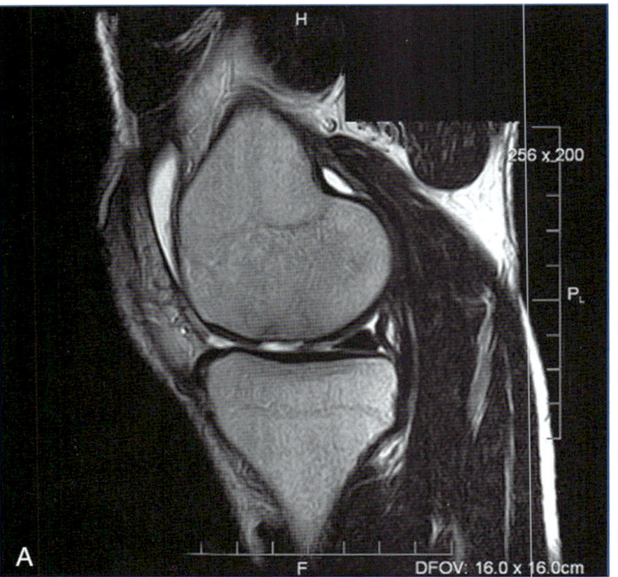

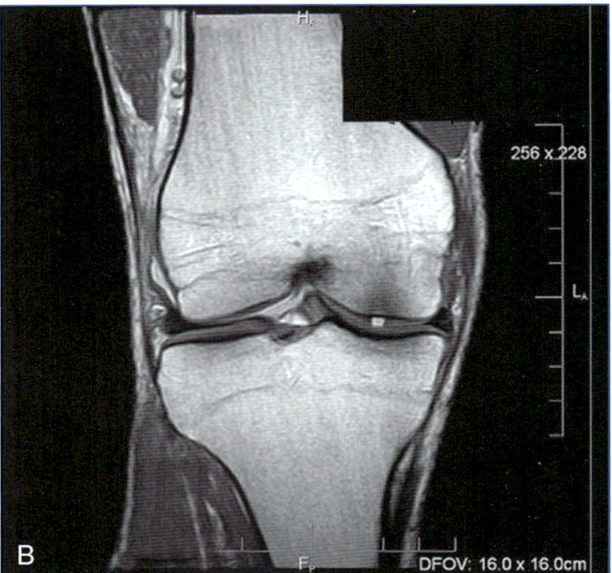

Figure 1 Sagittal (**A**) and coronal (**B**) T1-weighted MRIs of a 37-year-old man with medial-side knee pain and recurrent swelling. Note the greater size of the chondral lesion in the sagittal plane (**A**), a common finding.

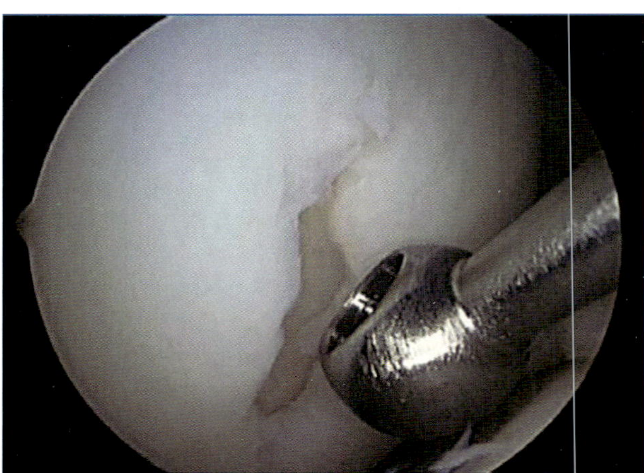

Figure 2 Arthroscopic view of the knee shown in Figure 1. The lesion is prepared for osteochondral autograft transplantation (OAT) by removing unstable chondral flaps and defining the size and shape of the defect.

involves only a one-stage procedure, is low cost, and carries no risk of disease transmission or immunologically mediated damage to the graft. Also, OAT is a minimally invasive procedure that can be performed through a small incision or even arthroscopically.

Case Presentation

History

A 37-year-old man presented with a history of a traumatic injury to the knee with subsequent medial knee pain, swelling, and significant activity limitation for more than 1 year. A focal chondral defect was discovered during the workup for ligamentous and meniscal injury. After an MRI was obtained to evaluate the chondral surfaces and assess the lesion size (Figure 1), the decision was made to perform osteochondral autograft transplantation (OAT). During the diagnostic portion of the arthroscopy, the lesion was identified and fully characterized. Free chondral flaps were débrided, and the subchondral bone was cleared of calcified cartilage (Figure 2). The focal chondral defect involved the weight-bearing portion of the medial femoral condyle. The lateral trochlear ridge was chosen as the donor site because it has been shown to be an acceptable match with respect to surface curvature and cartilage thickness for this

© 2011 *American Academy of Orthopaedic Surgeons*

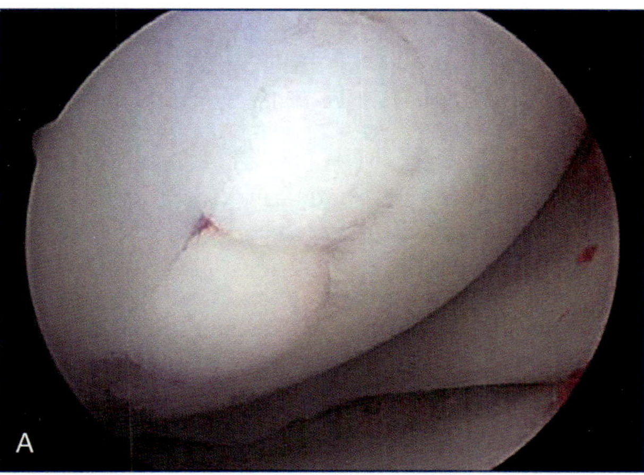

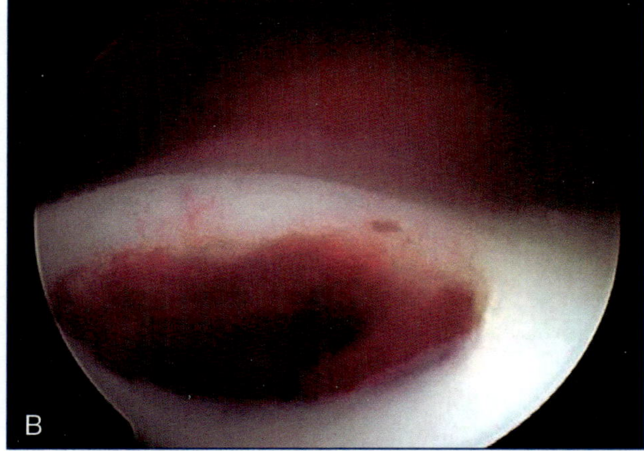

Figure 3 Arthroscopic views of the same knee shown in Figures 1 and 2. **A,** OAT, complete fill of the defect, and good restoration of articular surface contour are seen. **B,** The donor site from the lateral femoral trochlea is seen after plug harvest.

type of lesion. Trochlear defects are better matched by the cartilage in the concavity of the intercondylar notch. An OAT procedure was performed, and complete fill of the defect and good restoration of articular surface contour was achieved (Figure 3, A). The donor site was not backfilled (Figure 3, B). The patient was instructed on early knee range-of-motion exercises and restricted to non–weight-bearing ambulation for the first 6 weeks. Knee range of motion was evaluated 2 weeks after surgery, at the first postoperative visit. At 6 weeks after surgery, the patient was advanced to full weight bearing, and strengthening and range-of-motion exercises were continued for the next 6 weeks.

Current Problem

On subsequent visits to the clinic, the patient reported persistent knee pain. Physical examination revealed a mild knee effusion with a knee range of motion of 0° to 130°. There was no pain with patellar tracking or attempted lateral subluxation, but the patient did have crepitus with translation of the patella over the lateral aspect of the trochlear groove in the area of the donor site. The patient was encouraged to continue quadriceps strengthening as part of a home exercise program.

Donor-site morbidity can be an insidious pitfall of OAT. During OAT procedures, cylindrical transplants are harvested from the areas of the femoral condyles and trochlea that bear less weight, and the harvest sites routinely remain empty. Normally, natural healing processes originating in the cellular elements of the subchondral bone marrow result in fibrocartilage coverage of these harvest sites. These donor sites are filled by cancellous bone in 4 weeks and are covered by initial repair tissue in 6 weeks; fibrocartilage coverage develops within 8 to 12 weeks.

In a case report, LaPrade and Botker[1] identified two patients with pain and mechanical symptoms due to fibrocartilage hypertrophy (**Figure 4**) at the graft harvest site. Both patients were treated with abrasion of the overgrowth, and one required grafting of the site with allograft plugs. Many outcomes studies report minimal effects from graft harvest; however, true assessment of the contribution of donor-site morbidity to long-term symptoms is challenging in the injured knee. Reddy et al[2] evaluated donor-site morbidity in 15 patients treated with OAT for talar defects with grafts harvested from the ipsilateral asymptomatic knee. In the 11 patients available for follow-up, the average Lysholm knee score was 81, with 5 excellent, 2 good, and 4 poor results. One patient had patellar instability that was treated

© 2011 American Academy of Orthopaedic Surgeons

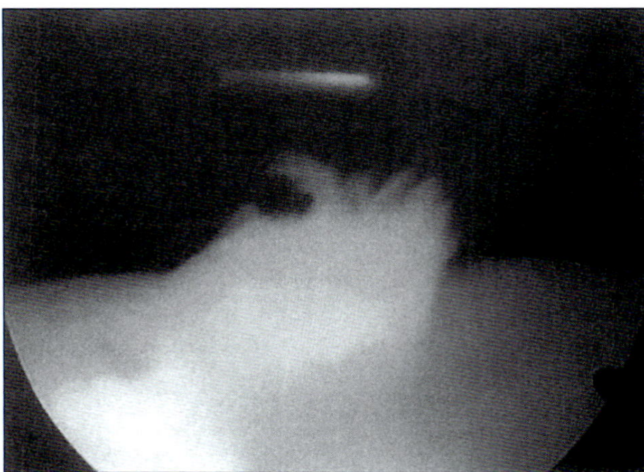

Figure 4 Arthroscopic view of the same knee shown in Figures 1 through 3 shows the donor site, where a 3.5-mm plug was harvested. Note hypertrophic fibrocartilage scar tissue at the superior aspect of the lateral trochlear groove.

with lateral retinacular release and tibial tubercle osteotomy. In contrast, Iwasaki et al[3] studied 11 competitive athletes treated with OAT for capitellar osteochondritis dissecans and found minimal knee symptoms from ipsilateral graft harvest. All patients returned to their previous level of competitive sport, and Lysholm and International Knee Documentation Committee scores were reported as excellent and normal, respectively, in all participants. Hangody and Füles[4] reported minimal long-term issues from graft harvest for the treatment of talar osteochondral defects. Knee pain from the graft harvest resolved in 6 weeks for 95% of the patients; by 1 year, 98% of knees were asymptomatic from the plug harvest. Because of the variability in donor-site symptoms after graft harvest, potential issues should be discussed with patients before surgery, with particular attention paid to anterior knee pain and mechanical symptoms from cartilage overgrowth.

Case Management and Outcome

The 37-year-old patient described at the opening of this chapter experienced continued pain and swelling of the knee. At 11 months after the OAT procedure, an MRI was obtained. The results were unremarkable. The decision was made to perform a diagnostic arthroscopy of the left knee to examine the donor grafting areas because of the pain and persistent crepitus on physical examination. The articular cartilage surfaces of the patella, medial and lateral femoral condyles, and medial and lateral tibial condyles were normal. The lateral aspect of the superior trochlear groove from which the grafts were taken had a large hypertrophic scar mound over two donor sites. A shaver was used to débride the area of hypertrophic fibrocartilage scar tissue to a flush stable rim. The patient was placed on crutches postoperatively for a 2-week period and then underwent rehabilitation. At the 2-year follow-up after arthroscopy, the patient had a full range of motion and no pain in the left knee with normal activity. Physical examination revealed no crepitus over the previous donor areas.

Other Complications: Incongruity

Overall congruity and contact pressure are better when fewer plugs are used for a circular defect.[5] In an experimental model, Hurtig et al[6] presented results of the treatment of a 15-mm defect with various combinations of grafts ranging from 2.7 to 6.5 mm in diameter. The researchers found significant cartilage loss and higher failure rates of small grafts due to their intrinsic fragility. The 4.5- and 6.5-mm grafts had intact cartilage at 90 days, with well-adherent mature connective tissue in interstices. Smaller plugs may be able to fill irregular defects with possibly less donor-site morbidity. Smaller grafts are more fragile; however, they have lower pullout strength, and technically they are more difficult to harvest and insert.[7] Larger-diameter grafts have increased graft stability. Hangody et al[8] suggested that a combination of 6.5- and 8.5-mm grafts may result in better outcomes than smaller grafts.

Other studies investigating the effect of incongruity of graft height on contact pressure suggest that plugs should be placed flush to the surrounding articular cartilage at the time of initial implantation.[9] Pearce et al[10] confirmed that deliberately proud grafts in a sheep model became flush with surround-

© 2011 American Academy of Orthopaedic Surgeons

ing cartilage. However, the authors also demonstrated persistent clefts at the margins, poor bony incorporation, subchondral cavitation, and fibroplasias. Indentation testing and contact pressure studies suggest that surface congruity plays an important role in avoiding early graft degeneration.

Strategies to Minimize Complications

Indications for OAT include a focal chondral defect without evidence of diffuse osteoarthritis and defect size typically limited to 1 to 4 cm^2.[11] Guettler et al[12] showed that rim stresses increase significantly with lesions greater than 10 mm in diameter. Because available donor-site material is limited, larger lesions may be amenable to allograft plug transfer. Con-comitant injuries affecting joint stability or mechanical axis alignment should be addressed at the time of surgery. Failure to correct these underlying issues may compromise plug survival and ultimate surgical outcomes. Although most OAT procedures are performed for femoral condyle defects, other applications include transfer to the patella, femoral trochlea, and tibia, and the use of plugs to secure unstable osteochondritis dissecans lesions. Contraindications include infection, tumor, degenerative joint disease, rheumatoid arthritis, and patient age greater than 50 years.

Several donor sites are available for graft harvest in the knee, and several variables should be considered before graft procurement. The medial and lateral trochlear regions and the medial and lateral aspects of the intercondylar notch are the most commonly used. These regions of the femur provide good-quality graft tissue from areas with low-weight-bearing characteristics. Donor sites may be accessed successfully through open or arthroscopic means. Because plugs should be harvested perpendicular to the surrounding chondral surface to decrease the risk of surface incongruity after transfer, harvest should focus on proper graft procurement rather than strict adherence to a single surgical approach or portal. Sites vary with respect to cartilage thickness, quality of surface curvature match, potential for donor-site morbidity, and accessibility. Although all are relatively non–weight bearing, several studies have shown that all sites experience some load during knee motion. The medial trochlea has less contact pressure than the lateral trochlea, and pressure values decrease as one moves distally along the lateral trochlea.[13] Guettler et al[14] noted no significant increase in these contact pressures with the harvest of a 5-mm graft plug from the lateral femoral trochlea. Because native cartilage thickness is directly proportional to the load across the region of the joint, it is not surprising that multiple studies have found that the low-weight-bearing areas used as donor sites have thinner cartilage than the recipient site. By using CT arthrography, Thaunat et al[15] showed that the lateral intercondylar notch has the thinnest cartilage of the commonly used donor sites. In a cadaver study, Ahmad et al[13] showed that the medial and lateral trochlea best matched the surface curvature of the condyles, and the concavity of the intercondylar notch best matched central trochlear defects. Bartz et al[5] reported similar findings, with medial and lateral trochlear sites showing superior surface match characteristics compared with the intercondylar notch, particularly with grafts larger than 6 mm in diameter. Graft harvest can result in marginal cell death, and minimizing the trauma to the plug is critical for maximizing cell viability after the transfer. Early techniques involved harvesting the plug with a power trephine, which led to unacceptable levels of chondrocyte loss.[16] Current protocols use a punch to obtain the plug, resulting in better protection of marginal chondrocytes in the graft tissue.

Multiple variables influence the quality of the transferred plug and affect the integrity and performance of the graft material. Just as harvest technique can affect chondrocyte viability, so too can the method of delivery. Borazjani et al[17] showed that the impaction of the graft into the recipient socket decreased cell survival, but they did not compare impaction with continuous-pressure delivery methods in that study. Because postoperative motion is imperative, a premium is placed on the stability of the transferred plug. Studies have shown that plugs of greater diameter are more stable than smaller plugs because of increased frictional force at the graft-socket interface.[18] Additionally, plugs that rest on the bottom of the recipient socket show increased stability with early motion.[19] Single plugs are more stable than multiple plugs; however, the pattern of mosaic reconstruction does not appear to affect ini-

© 2011 *American Academy of Orthopaedic Surgeons*

tial graft stability. Careful attention should be paid to proper retrieval and insertion of the graft because security of the plug also can be affected by surgical technique. Duchow et al[18] showed that removal and reinsertion during transplantation decreased plug stability, as did toggling of the harvesting tool during graft extraction from the donor site.

The height of the graft and angle of the chondral surface of the graft relative to the surrounding articular cartilage also influence the quality of the chondral repair. Plugs delivered flush or slightly recessed compared with the surrounding surface have contact pressures similar to that of native cartilage, whereas grafts left proud cause an increase in pressure at the articular surface and show poorer integration with the surrounding cartilage.[20] Excessive recession also can be detrimental. In an ovine model, Huang et al[21] showed that grafts recessed 1 mm or less demonstrated remodeling potential with cartilage thickening and improvement of surface incongruity, whereas plugs recessed 2 mm or more had increased cell death and surface fibrillation. Plugs should be harvested and delivered perpendicular to the surrounding cartilage surface to decrease the contact pressure during weight-bearing activity. Angled harvest or delivery results in a high and a low side of the graft, causing a surface incongruity that can compromise results of the procedure. In the event of an angled graft, contact pressures are minimized by orienting the graft so that all portions of the graft are slightly recessed. Placing the angled graft with the high side elevated above the surrounding cartilage results in an increase in local contact pressure and should be avoided. Despite close attention to surgical technique, the potential remains for harvest or delivery of the graft at nonperpendicular angles. In an evaluation of surgical videos from index procedures, Barber and Chow[22] showed that 50% of plugs were inserted 10° from perpendicular to the chondral surface. Repeat arthroscopy of these knees showed no evidence of problems with integration or resurfacing issues, and compromise of clinical outcomes was not observed. Second-look arthroscopy and tissue biopsies showed that viable chondrocytes and osteocytes as well as hyaline cartilage remain at the graft site.[22]

The transferred osteochondral plug demonstrates time-dependent changes in its mechanical properties. Immediately after transfer, the plug shows stiffness, surface integrity, and thickness similar to the harvest site. Studies have shown that some of these properties are compromised in the early stages after transplantation but improve as the graft incorporates into the surrounding bone and cartilage interface.[23] These findings support the current approach to limited weight bearing in the immediate postoperative period. Despite good bony integration, plug viability, and restoration of surface contour, a cleft frequently persists at the interface of the plug cartilage and the articular surface surrounding the recipient socket. The effects of this residual cleft on long-term plug survival and clinical results have not been established.

References

1. LaPrade RF, Botker JC: Donor-site morbidity after osteochondral autograft transfer procedures. *Arthroscopy* 2004;20(7):e69-e73.
2. Reddy S, Pedowitz DI, Parekh SG, Sennett BJ, Okereke E: The morbidity associated with osteochondral harvest from asymptomatic knees for the treatment of osteochondral lesions of the talus. *Am J Sports Med* 2007;35(1):80-85.
3. Iwasaki N, Kato H, Kamishima T, Suenaga N, Minami A: Donor site evaluation after autologous osteochondral mosaicplasty for cartilaginous lesions of the elbow joint. *Am J Sports Med* 2007;35(12):2096-2100.
4. Hangody L, Füles P: Autologous osteochondral mosaicplasty for the treatment of full-thickness defects of weight-bearing joints: Ten years of experimental and clinical experience. *J Bone Joint Surg Am* 2003;85-A (Suppl 2):25-32.
5. Bartz RL, Kamaric E, Noble PC, Lintner D, Bocell J: Topographic matching of selected donor and recipient sites for osteochondral autografting of the articular surface of the femoral condyles. *Am J Sports Med* 2001;29(2):207-212.
6. Hurtig MB, Novak K, McPherson R, et al: Osteochondral dowel transplantation for repair of focal defects in the knee: An outcome study using an ovine model. *Vet Surg* 1998;27(1):5-16.
7. Kordás G, Szabó JS, Hangody L: The effect of drill-hole length on the primary stability of osteochondral grafts in mosaicplasty. *Orthopedics* 2005;28(4):401-404.
8. Hangody L, Dobos J, Baló E, Pánics G, Hangody LR, Berkes I: Clinical experiences with autologous osteochondral mosaicplasty in an athletic population: A 17-year prospective multicenter study. *Am J Sports Med* 2010;38(6):1125-1133.

© 2011 American Academy of Orthopaedic Surgeons

9. Hurtig M, Pearce S, Warren S, Kalra M, Miniaci A: Arthroscopic mosaic arthroplasty in the equine third carpal bone. *Vet Surg* 2001;30(3):228-239.
10. Pearce SG, Hurtig MB, Clarnette R, Kalra MS, Cowan B, Miniaci A: An investigation of 2 techniques for optimizing joint surface congruency using multiple cylindrical osteochondral autografts. *Arthroscopy* 2001;17(1): 50-55.
11. Hangody L, Feczkó P, Bartha L, Bodó G, Kish G: Mosaicplasty for the treatment of articular defects of the knee and ankle. *Clin Orthop Relat Res* 2001(391 Suppl):S328-S336.
12. Guettler JH, Demetropoulos CK, Yang KH, Jurist KA: Osteochondral defects in the human knee: Influence of defect size on cartilage rim stress and load redistribution to surrounding cartilage. *Am J Sports Med* 2004;32(6):1451-1458.
13. Ahmad CS, Cohen ZA, Levine WN, Ateshian GA, Mow VC: Biomechanical and topographic considerations for autologous osteochondral grafting in the knee. *Am J Sports Med* 2001;29(2):201-206.
14. Guettler JH, Demetropoulos CK, Yang KH, Jurist KA: Dynamic evaluation of contact pressure and the effects of graft harvest with subsequent lateral release at osteochondral donor sites in the knee. *Arthroscopy* 2005;21(6):715-720.
15. Thaunat M, Couchon S, Lunn J, Charrois O, Fallet L, Beaufils P: Cartilage thickness matching of selected donor and recipient sites for osteochondral autografting of the medial femoral condyle. *Knee Surg Sports Traumatol Arthrosc* 2007;15(4):381-386.
16. Evans PJ, Miniaci A, Hurtig MB: Manual punch versus power harvesting of osteochondral grafts. *Arthroscopy* 2004;20(3):306-310.
17. Borazjani BH, Chen AC, Bae WC, et al: Effect of impact on chondrocyte viability during insertion of human osteochondral grafts. *J Bone Joint Surg Am* 2006;88(9):1934-1943.
18. Duchow J, Hess T, Kohn D: Primary stability of press-fit-implanted osteochondral grafts: Influence of graft size, repeated insertion, and harvesting technique. *Am J Sports Med* 2000;28(1):24-27.
19. Kock NB, Van Susante JL, Buma P, Van Kampen A, Verdonschot N: Press-fit stability of an osteochondral autograft: Influence of different plug length and perfect depth alignment. *Acta Orthop* 2006;77(3):422-428.
20. Koh JL, Kowalski A, Lautenschlager E: The effect of angled osteochondral grafting on contact pressure: A biomechanical study. *Am J Sports Med* 2006;34(1): 116-119.
21. Huang FS, Simonian PT, Norman AG, Clark JM: Effects of small incongruities in a sheep model of osteochondral autografting. *Am J Sports Med* 2004;32(8): 1842-1848.
22. Barber FA, Chow JC: Arthroscopic chondral osseous autograft transplantation (COR procedure) for femoral defects. *Arthroscopy* 2006;22(1):10-16.
23. Nakaji N, Fujioka H, Nagura I, et al: The structural properties of an osteochondral cylinder graft-recipient construct on autologous osteochondral transplantation. *Arthroscopy* 2006;22(4):422-427.

© 2011 American Academy of Orthopaedic Surgeons

Chapter 3

Osteochondral Allografts

William Bugbee, MD

Case Presentation

A 20-year-old man sustained an isolated injury to the lateral femoral condyle of the left knee (**Figure 1**). After failure of nonsurgical management, he underwent arthroscopic evaluation and chondroplasty. He continued to have symptoms despite further nonsurgical management. Because of the size and osseous involvement of the lesion, 1 year after initial injury he underwent osteochondral allografting of the lateral femoral condyle using a single plug. The patient had an unremarkable initial postoperative course and returned to normal activities. (The patient was not involved in competitive high-impact sports.) At 9 months after the allograft procedure, he developed recurrent pain and mechanical symptoms with weight bearing. The recurrent symptoms did not occur after acute injury or trauma but were more gradual in onset. Clinical evaluation revealed a small knee joint effusion, focal tenderness over the lateral femoral condyle, no meniscal signs, and a stable knee with normal limb alignment. Imaging studies including plain radiographs and MRI demonstrated cystic degeneration, fragmentation, and collapse of the allograft (**Figure 2**).

Discussion

Osteochondral allografts have emerged as an important treatment option for restoration of diseased or damaged articular cartilage. Because of their versatility in managing simple and complex problems, the use of allografts in clini-

---

Dr. Bugbee or an immediate family member serves as a board member, owner, officer, or committee member of the American Academy of Orthopaedic Surgeons Biologic Implants Committee and Advanced Biohealing; has received royalties from Smith & Nephew and Zimmer; serves as a paid consultant to or is an employee of Arthrex, DePuy, Smith & Nephew, Zimmer, and the Joint Restoration Foundation; and has received research or institutional support from the Orthopaedic Research and Education Foundation.

© 2011 American Academy of Orthopaedic Surgeons

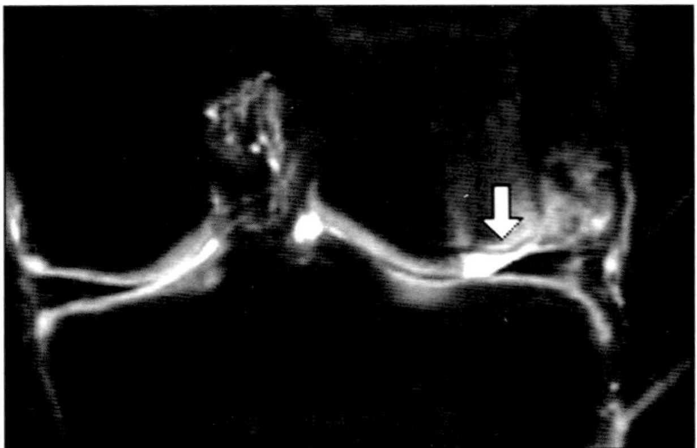

Figure 1 T2-weighted MRI of a 20-year-old man with a chondral lesion of the lateral femoral condyle. Note the change in signal intensity in the subchondral bone (arrow).

cal practice has expanded. Typical indications for osteochondral allografts in cartilage repair include primary treatment of large chondral lesions and revision of lesions previously treated with other repair modalities (eg, microfracture, osteochondral autografting, or autologous chondrocyte implantation). In addition, allografts have been used in treating more challenging osteochondral lesions such as osteochondritis dissecans, osteonecrosis, and periarticular trauma deformity. An extensive body of literature exists describing the scientific basis, technical aspects, and clinical outcome of osteochondral allografting.[1] As with other cartilage repair techniques, clinical success (and failure) depends on patient selection, surgical technique, and the biologic response of the host. However, osteochondral allografts also have

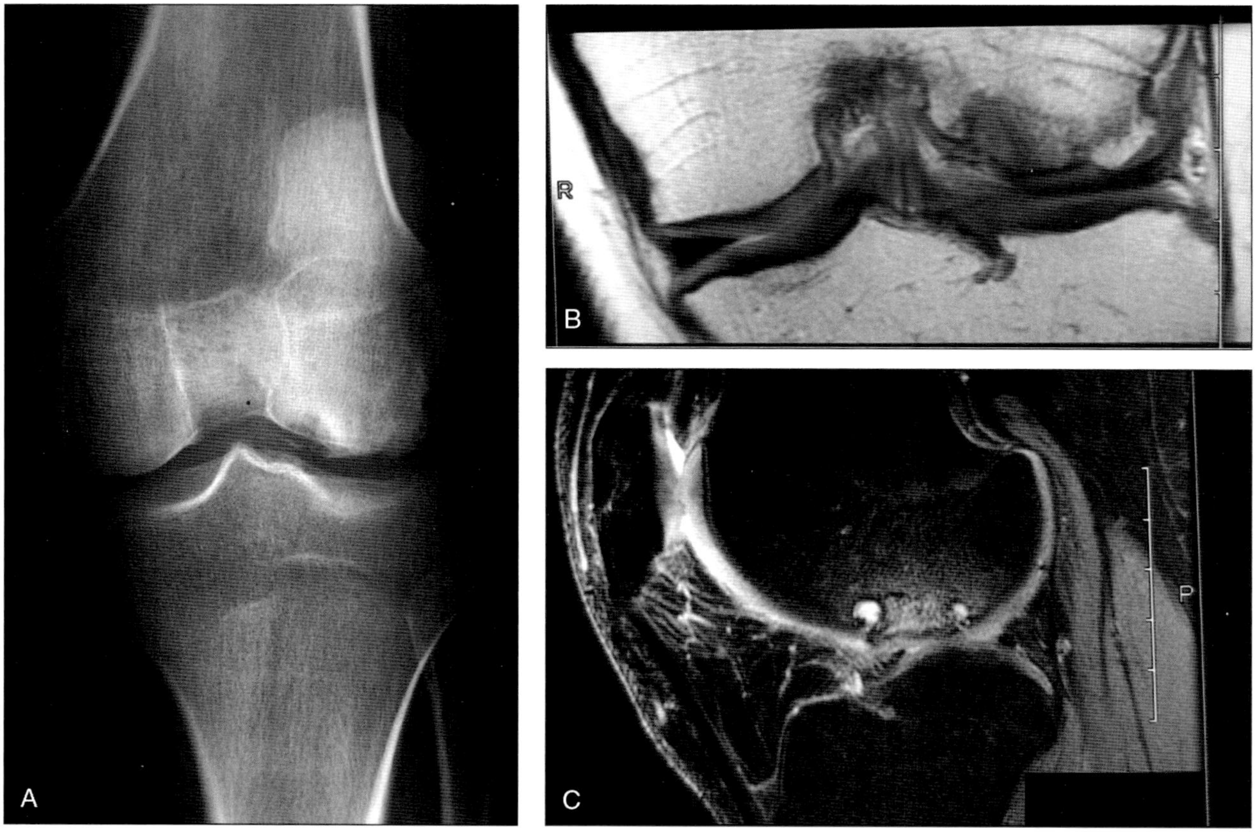

Figure 2 Images of the patient in Figure 1 obtained 1 year after he underwent an allograft procedure. **A,** AP radiograph demonstrates fragmentation of subchondral bone and radiolucency in the medial aspect of the allograft. **B,** Coronal MRI demonstrates incongruity of the subchondral plate and cyst formation. **C,** Sagittal MRI shows subchondral cyst formation at the margins of the allograft.

© 2011 American Academy of Orthopaedic Surgeons

unique features that are important to consider when evaluating potential failure. In particular, because an osteochondral allograft is a composite of two tissue components, bone and cartilage, either of these can be implicated in graft failure. However, in my experience, complications associated with the osseous portion of the graft are far more common than complications associated with the chondral component. Transplantation of allograft tissue also includes the inherent risk of disease transmission from the graft to the recipient, as well as the potential for immunologic response by the host to the donor tissue.

Incidence of Complications

The incidence of complications in osteochondral allografting is difficult to quantify because most published studies involve heterogeneous treatment groups, relatively small cohorts, and short-term follow-up. For example, in the treatment of posttraumatic arthritis or secondary osteoarthrosis, graft "failure," defined as conversion to joint arthroplasty, is as high as 28% at 5 to 15 years.[2] In reality, many of these patients did not have graft failure, but rather had progression of osteoarthritis or unresolved symptoms that led to reoperation. Conversely, graft survivorship in the treatment of focal femoral condyle lesions is greater than 90% in all published studies, with a reoperation rate less than 10%.[3-6] **Table 1** summarizes our experience at Scripps Clinic and the University of California, San Diego, over the last 27 years, where 515 patients have undergone 576 knee allograft procedures. Of those, 328 patients (354 knees) were available for minimum 2-year follow-up and 187 patients (222 knees) were not available (59 patients were less than 2 years from surgery). Mean follow-up was 86 months (range, 24 to 309 months). Seventy-two knees (20%) underwent a reoperation that included removal or revision of the allograft and were defined as clinical failures. The 72 failures included 41 total knee arthroplasties, 23 revision allografts, 4 partial knee arthroplasties, 2 patellectomies, and 2 knee fusions. The mean time to failure was 40 months (range, 3 to 165 months). Survivorship was 82% at 5 years, 72% at 10 years, and 70% at 25 years. Failure rates by diagnosis are shown in **Table 2**. Factors correlated with increased failure were female sex, age more than 40 years, and a large graft area (>10 cm²). Consequently, factors that correlated with success were graft area less than 10 cm² and age less than 30 years.

Although these data reflect a tertiary referral experience, including both simple focal lesions and complex salvage cases with large or multiple grafts, they underscore the relatively high reoperation rates that have been reported for allografting, as well as other cartilage repair procedures. Most surgeons use allografts for simple focal lesions of the femoral condyle and therefore should expect much lower reoperation rates (5% to 15%) during early or midterm follow-up.

TABLE 1 Patient Characteristics and Allograft Details (N = 354 knees)[a]

Variable	Value
Mean age (y)	34 (SD, 11.8; range, 14-68)
Male sex	53.1
Diagnosis (%)	
Osteochondritis dissecans	26.8
Degenerative chondral lesion	22.6
Traumatic chondral injury	14.7
Osteoarthritis	12.4
Osteonecrosis	9.3
Fracture	7.1
Failed osteochondral allograft	7.1
Previous surgery on affected joint	90.7
Mean number of previous surgeries	2.6 (SD, 1.8; range, 1-13)
Graft location (%)	
Femoral condyle (medial)	35.3
Femoral condyle (lateral)	18.4
Tibial plateau (medial)	1.1
Tibial plateau (lateral)	2.5
Patella	7.6
Trochlea	5.4
Two locations	26.3
Three locations	3.4
Mean number of grafts	1.5 (SD, 0.7; range, 1-4)
Mean total graft area (cm²)	10.1 (SD, 7.0; range, 1.2-57.5)

[a] Procedures performed at Scripps Clinic, La Jolla, CA, and the University of California, San Diego, from 1983 to 2009.

© 2011 American Academy of Orthopaedic Surgeons

TABLE 2 Allograft Failure Rates by Diagnosis (N = 72)[a]

Diagnosis	Number of Knees	Failure Rate (%)
Osteochondritis dissecans	11	15.3
Degenerative chondral lesion	14	19.4
Traumatic chondral injury	7	9.7
Osteoarthritis	21	29.2
Osteonecrosis	5	6.9
Fracture	6	8.4
Failed osteochondral allograft	8	11.1

[a] Procedures performed at Scripps Clinic, La Jolla, CA, and the University of California, San Diego, from 1983 to 2009.

Recognizing Complications

Complications associated with osteochondral allografting of the knee can be loosely classified into two categories: those directly related to the allograft (nonunion, fracture, collapse, or chondrolysis/delamination), and those not necessarily related to the allograft itself (infection, effusion, arthrofibrosis, and persistent pain).

Infection

Infection can manifest as cellulitis, wound infection, or deep joint-space infection. As with any intra-articular procedure, the threshold for reoperation should be low. The unique issue associated with allografting is determining whether the infection is graft related and determining if the graft should be retained or removed. Although serious infections associated with osteochondral allografting have been reported,[7] no allograft-associated infections occurred in the Scripps series described above. This is likely due to strict adherence to donor recovery and processing, copious lavage of the graft before insertion, and the relatively healthy population of recipient patients. It should be noted that traditional or typical surgical-site infections (eg, *Staphylococcus aureus*) are statistically far more common than infections caused by allograft contamination (often unusual organisms such as clostridial species). Any infection thought to be related to an allograft should be reported to the tissue bank providing the graft.

Stiffness and Arthrofibrosis

Postoperative stiffness and arthrofibrosis are not unique to allograft surgery and can be managed similarly to other postoperative situations. Risk factors include previous history, poor preoperative motion, a multiply operated joint, extensive surgery or postoperative management requiring limited early range of motion, or poor rehabilitation effort. Manipulation under anesthesia may be necessary if modification of rehabilitation protocols is unsuccessful.

Prolonged Effusion

My colleagues and I noted a persistent joint effusion in a small number of patients. The etiology of this phenomenon is under investigation and may be multifactorial. In some cases, overexuberant postoperative activity may be implicated, but other cases may be due to biologic or immunologic response to the allograft. Patients with significant preoperative effusions often have persistent postoperative effusions; in this situation, the underlying disease state of the joint may have led to "synovial activation" that requires time to resolve. Patients with grafts of the patellofemoral joint seem to be particularly prone to effusions. The recommendation is for observation once infection has been ruled out. Synovial fluid analysis, including cell count, differential, and crystal analysis, should be performed if the effusion persists. Rheumatologic workup can be considered, as there is a possibility of an inflammatory condition unrelated to the allograft. Likewise, a secondary joint pathology such as a meniscal tear, loose body, or chondral flap may be present and should be ruled out.

Persistent Pain

Persistent postoperative pain without obvious cause can be frustrating. In many joints undergoing allografting, multiple pathologies in addition to the articular lesion are present. Furthermore, these patients have often had multiple previous surgeries and longstanding pain. This underscores the importance of patient selection and careful verification that the source of pain or symptoms correlates with the lesion

© 2011 American Academy of Orthopaedic Surgeons

being treated. In complex cases, a diagnostic anesthetic injection is helpful, not only as part of preoperative evaluation but also postoperatively, when the source of pain is enigmatic. Interpretation of imaging studies such as MRI should be done with caution, as most allografts have an abnormal appearance and many radiologists are unfamiliar with this condition. In the absence of symptoms attributable to the allograft (discussed below), the most common causes are new or secondary lesions or progression of joint disease into established osteoarthritis. Diagnostic and/or therapeutic arthroscopy may be indicated in this setting.

Allograft-Related Complications

Because of the unique nature of the osteochondral allograft technique, complications associated with the allograft itself are perhaps the most important to recognize and treat appropriately. Allograft-associated complications can be divided into three subsets: problems with healing (delayed union or nonunion); late graft fragmentation, fracture, or collapse; and chondrolysis or chondral delamination. Nonunion or delayed union is extremely rare with modern surgical techniques using instrumentation for plugs or dowels rather than onlay or inlay shell-grafting techniques.[8] Conversely, cases of chondrolysis or chondral delamination are now seen more commonly. This may be the result of the deleterious effects of prolonged graft storage necessary for commercial distribution of allografts alone,[9] or in combination with the unfortunate surgical maneuver of forceful impaction of the allograft during insertion, which has been shown to cause chondrocyte death.[10]

By far the most common entity is late graft osseous failure. This may take the form of cystic degeneration, fragmentation, fracture, or collapse. Failure of the osteochondral allograft is usually manifested in acute or insidious onset of symptoms very similar to the original presenting condition. This may be purely mechanical, with catching, locking, or swelling without significant pain, or recurrent focal pain, particularly with weight bearing. The timing of allograft failure is variable. Although it is unusual to reoperate on the allograft within the first year, prodromal symptoms such as persistent soreness or effusion may present within months of return to weight bearing or progression to higher impact activity. More commonly, the patient has an excellent early result, but new symptoms develop 1 or more years after the allograft surgery. At Scripps, we have seen primary allograft failure (graft collapse or fragmentation) any time from 1 to 14 years after surgery. Recognizing failure of the allograft is usually straightforward, but it may take some time to exclude other causes of symptoms. The general clinical picture of a failing allograft is remarkably similar to that of osteochondritis dissecans or osteonecrosis, for those familiar with these conditions. Serial high-quality radiographs at 3- to 6-month intervals usually show subtle or obvious changes in the osseous portion of the graft. MRI can be helpful as well, with the caveat that well-functioning allografts may have very abnormal signal on MRI.[11] Key findings include the presence of fluid at the host-graft interface, cyst formation (although small solitary cysts are common in well-functioning grafts), disruption and irregularity of the subchondral plate, or frank fragmentation and collapse. Very rarely does graft failure manifest with early complete loss of chondral tissue. Diagnostic arthroscopy may show softening of the graft, loose bodies or attached fragments, or thinning or fibrillation of cartilage. Because the initial pathology is usually osseous and not chondral (akin to osteochondritis dissecans or osteonecrosis), the articular surface may appear healthy and pristine. Individuals at higher risk of failure include those with larger grafts that support a greater percentage of joint load or patients with multiple grafts, each having an independent risk of failure. The volume of the allograft appears to be correlated with failure, with larger allografts more likely to become problematic. This is likely due to the inherent biology of allograft bone healing. Many studies have shown limitations of creeping substitution and revascularization of allograft bone.[12] For this reason, I tend to minimize the volume of bone transplanted, unless osseous reconstruction is necessary. Most femoral condyle lesions can be reconstructed with graft of a combined (bone and cartilage) thickness of 5 to 8 mm. Although unproven in clinical studies, patients with untreated limb malalignment, instability, or profound meniscus deficiency may be at higher risk of failure because of the potential for high load-

© 2011 American Academy of Orthopaedic Surgeons

ing patterns being placed on the allograft. Conversely, I have not seen any correlation between graft failure and return to high-demand sports. This is an area of considerable controversy and study, as the use of relatively high-risk surgical procedures such as osteotomy and mensical transplantation is often recommended with allografting, and the counseling of patients regarding postoperative activity is fraught with uncertainly because of limited data. Retrieval studies on failed osteochondral allografts provide some insight into the biology of fresh osteochondral allografts and mechanisms of failure.[13,14]

Managing Allograft Failure

Managing allograft failure may include observation with routine clinical and radiographic follow-up. This may be appropriate if symptoms are modest and the patient is functioning well or had changed activity to accommodate dysfunction. Often, knee scores in patients with signs of allograft failure are not "excellent" but are better than they were preoperatively. This is often true of patients treated with allografts in salvage situations, with the only other option being arthroplasty. In these patients, the graft failure may be superimposed on global decline of the joint in general (osteoarthrosis).

Diagnostic and therapeutic arthroscopy is often the first surgical treatment of patients with the presumed diagnosis of failed allograft. The arthroscopy helps define the failure mode and guide further treatment, or it may uncover other treatable pathology such as a meniscal tear or new chondral injury. Débridement or chondroplasty of the allograft may be useful and often leads to symptomatic relief. Arthroscopy is the most commonreoperationI have performed after allografting. Revision osteochondral allografting may be necessary in cases of symptomatic allograft failure. In most cases, the revision procedure follows the same general pattern and technique of a primary allograft procedure. Typically, the failed allograft lesion is not larger than the original defect and may, in fact, be smaller, as it is rare to have failure of the entire allograft. Occasionally, extension of chondral disease or new satellite lesions require consideration of more extensive grafting during the revision. Key points to consider when undertaking revision allografting include the following:

The root cause of the failure of the first procedure, such as uncorrected malalignment or technical error (excessive graft thickness, instability, incongruent fit, or inappropriate impaction during insertion), should be determined. Often, the initial allografting was performed well and no real "cause" other than failure of biologic incorporation can be determined.

The biologic or mechanical environment for the new graft should be improved. This includes attention to alignment and joint stability, prolonging the postoperative weight-bearing restrictions (up to 3 months), using thinner grafts with autografting of deeper cysts, and copious irrigation of the allograft to remove marrow elements before insertion. Gentle insertion forces placed on the graft with occasional use of fixation devices such as chondral darts (Arthrex, Naples, FL) or biocompression screws is preferred over high-impact techniques that may lead to graft damage. My experience suggests that nonunion of an allograft is far less common than healing of the allograft with subsequent collapse and fragmentation.

Revision allografting appears to have a success rate similar to that of primary allografting, which is related to patient and disease characteristics. Therefore, I consider revision allografting the procedure of choice in the treatment of allograft failure. Although my colleagues and I occasionally salvage failed allografts with unicompartmental or total joint arthroplasty, this is typically in the context of more complex salvage cases in older individuals who originally declined arthroplasty as a treatment of the original condition.

Preventing Complications

Preventing late graft failure can be problematic. Attention to the key points mentioned above (mechanical environment and technical factors) is important. However, some uncertainty remains, related to poorly understood biologic or immunologic factors that may play a role in some cases of late allograft failure.

© 2011 American Academy of Orthopaedic Surgeons

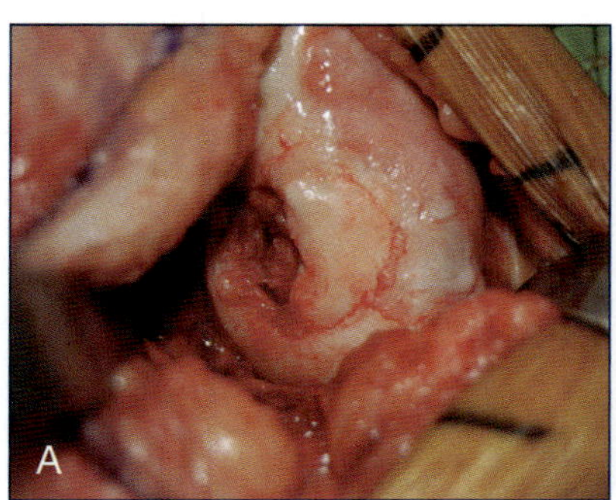

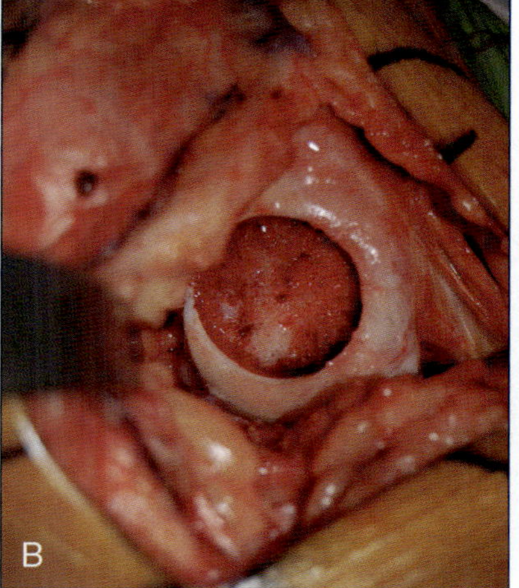

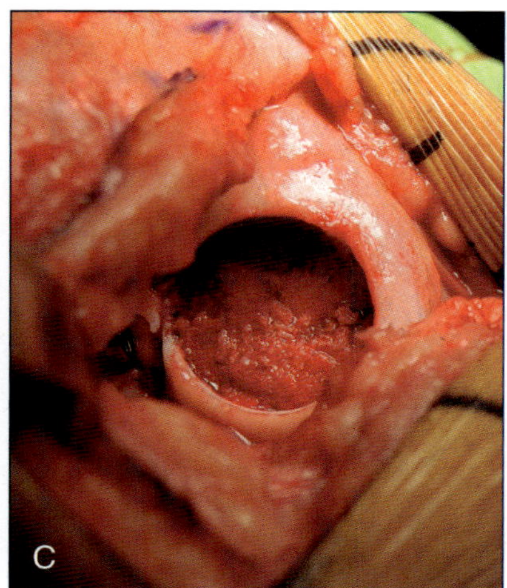

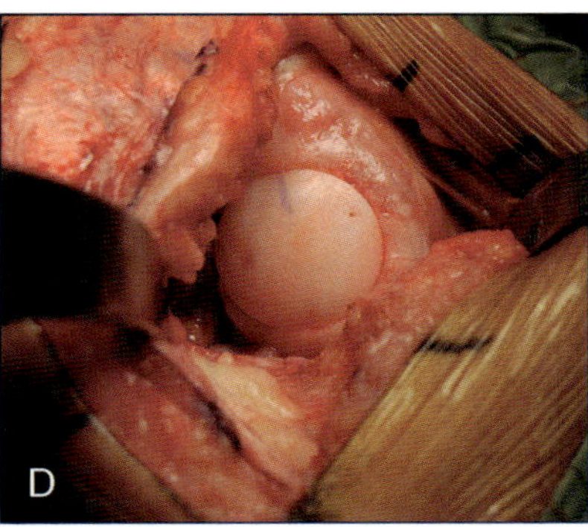

Figure 3 Intraoperative photographs of the knee of the patient shown in Figures 1 and 2, obtained during reoperation at 15 months after initial allograft procedure. **A,** Appearance of failed graft. Complete loss of the medial part of the graft with relative preservation of the lateral portion can be seen. **B,** The host condyle after preparatory reaming of failed allograft. Note the minimal depth of reaming and presence of subchondral cysts (seen in white), but relative preservation of healthy, bleeding bone. **C,** Bone grafting of the cysts has been performed and the site is ready for allograft implantation. Note that the size of the grafting site is only marginally larger than the original allograft. **D,** Completed implantation of the new allograft. The allograft is congruent with the surrounding articular surface and is fixed with two chondral darts.

Case Management

Fifteen months after the initial allografting procedure, the patient shown in **Figures 1** and **2** underwent revision osteochondral allografting with another plug allograft. Findings at surgery included fragmentation of the medial portion of the allograft with areas of subchondral cyst formation. Most of the allograft had healed to host bone, and the articular cartilage was intact (**Figure 3**, *A*). The revision procedure included bone grafting of small cysts in the host bone and implantation of an allograft of similar diameter to the original graft but thinner than the original (graft thickness, 7 to 8 mm) (**Figure 3**, *B* through *D*). The patient was maintained on toe-touch weight bearing for 8 weeks, followed by progressive weight bearing for an additional 8 weeks. Range of motion was not restricted. The patient had an uneventful recovery with resolution of symptoms by 6 months. Radiographs obtained at that time showed healing of the allograft (**Figure 4**).

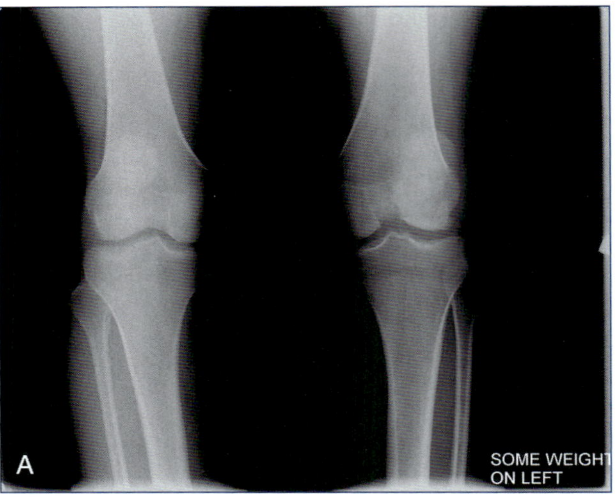

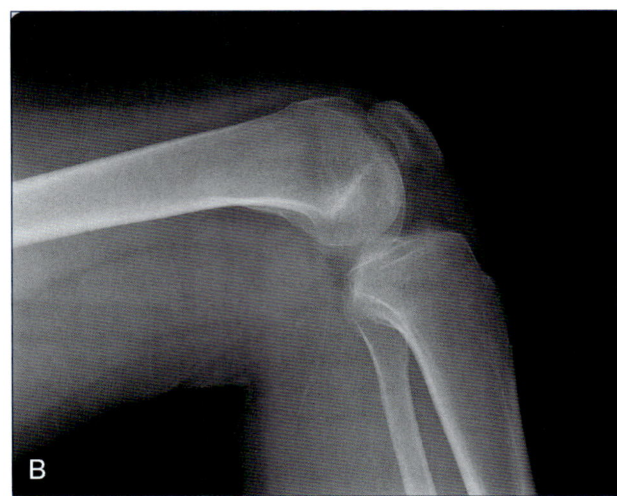

Figure 4 Weight-bearing AP (**A**) and lateral (**B**) radiographs of the knee of the patient shown in Figures 1 through 3 obtained 6 months after the revision allograft procedure. Note healing of the osseous interface and restoration of subchondral bone.

References

1. Görtz S, Bugbee WD: Allografts in articular cartilage repair. *J Bone Joint Surg Am* 2006;88(6):1374-1384.
2. Görtz S, De Young A, Bugbee WD: Paper 513: Fresh osteochondral allograft transplantation for biopolar cartilage lesions of the knee. *Annual Meeting Proceedings*. Rosemont, IL, American Academy of Orthopaedic Surgeons, 2009, p 784.
3. Williams RJ III, Ranawat AS, Potter HG, Carter T, Warren RF: Fresh stored allografts for the treatment of osteochondral defects of the knee. *J Bone Joint Surg Am* 2007;89(4):718-726.
4. McCulloch PC, Kang RW, Sobhy MH, Hayden JK, Cole BJ: Prospective evaluation of prolonged fresh osteochondral allograft transplantation of the femoral condyle: Minimum 2-year follow-up. *Am J Sports Med* 2007;35(3):411-420.
5. Emmerson BC, Görtz S, Jamali AA, Chung C, Amiel D, Bugbee WD: Fresh osteochondral allografting in the treatment of osteochondritis dissecans of the femoral condyle. *Am J Sports Med* 2007;35(6):907-914.
6. LaPrade RF, Botker J, Herzog M, Agel J: Refrigerated osteoarticular allografts to treat articular cartilage defects of the femoral condyles: A prospective outcomes study. *J Bone Joint Surg Am* 2009;91(4):805-811.
7. Tomford WW: Transmission of disease through transplantation of musculoskeletal allografts. *J Bone Joint Surg Am* 1995;77(11):1742-1754.
8. Bugbee W: Allograft osteochondral plugs, in Jackson DW, ed: *Reconstructive Knee Surgery*, ed 3. Philadelphia, PA, Lippincott Williams & Wilkins, 2008, pp 475-483.
9. Ball ST, Amiel D, Williams SK, et al: The effects of storage on fresh human osteochondral allografts. *Clin Orthop Relat Res* 2004(418):246-252.
10. Borazjani BH, Chen AC, Bae WC, et al: Effect of impact on chondrocyte viability during insertion of human osteochondral grafts. *J Bone Joint Surg Am* 2006;88(9):1934-1943.
11. Sirlin CB, Brossmann J, Boutin RD, et al: Shell osteochondral allografts of the knee: Comparison of mr imaging findings and immunologic responses. *Radiology* 2001;219(1):35-43.
12. Burchardt H: The biology of bone graft repair. *Clin Orthop Relat Res* 1983(174):28-42.
13. Kandel RA, Gross AE, Ganel A, McDermott AG, Langer F, Pritzker KP: Histopathology of failed osteoarticular shell allografts. *Clin Orthop Relat Res* 1985(197):103-110.
14. Williams SK, Amiel D, Ball ST, et al: Analysis of cartilage tissue on a cellular level in fresh osteochondral allograft retrievals. *Am J Sports Med* 2007;35(12):2022-2032.

© 2011 American Academy of Orthopaedic Surgeons

Chapter 4

Autologous Chondrocyte Implantation

Andreas H. Gomoll, MD

Introduction

Autologous chondrocyte implantation (ACI) with Carticel (Genzyme BioSurgery, Cambridge, MA) is a two-stage cartilage repair procedure using an arthrotomy for implantation of cultured autologous chondrocytes under a periosteal membrane cover.[1] In addition to carrying the risks of any open knee surgery, such as infection and arthrofibrosis, the procedure also is associated with several complications specific to ACI, such as graft delamination and hypertrophy.[2]

This chapter provides an overview of the most common complications associated with ACI and presents strategies for minimizing the risk of their occurrence, although the risk cannot be completely negated. In addition, it discusses how to recognize and treat complications when they occur despite the clinician's best efforts. Finally, setbacks are common during the rehabilitation process after ACI, and although they are not true complications, they can be very unsettling and frustrating to both the patient and health care providers. This chapter addresses how to modify rehabilitation to address such setbacks.

Case 1: Graft and Patch Hypertrophy

History

A 32-year-old man presented with a large cartilage defect of the trochlea. Nonsurgical measures had failed. He underwent uneventful treatment with ACI for a 6-cm^2 defect and concurrent tibial tubercle osteotomy. He followed the standard postoperative rehabilitation program and progressed steadily without significant setbacks.

Dr. Gomoll or an immediate family member is a member of a speakers' bureau or has made paid presentations on behalf of Arthrex and Genzyme; serves as a paid consultant to or is an employee of Genzyme; and has received research or institutional support from Genzyme and ConforMIS.

© 2011 American Academy of Orthopaedic Surgeons

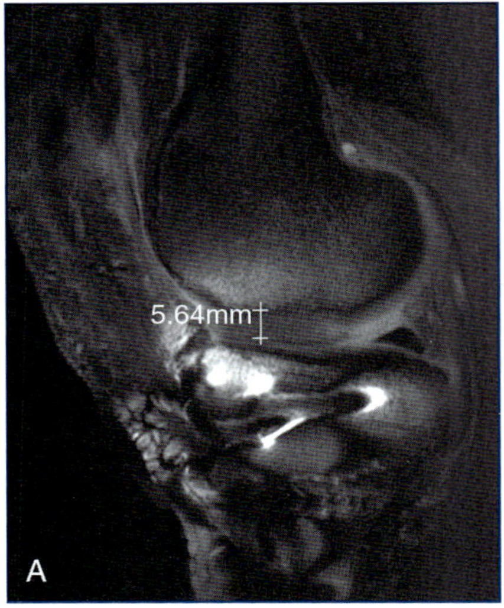

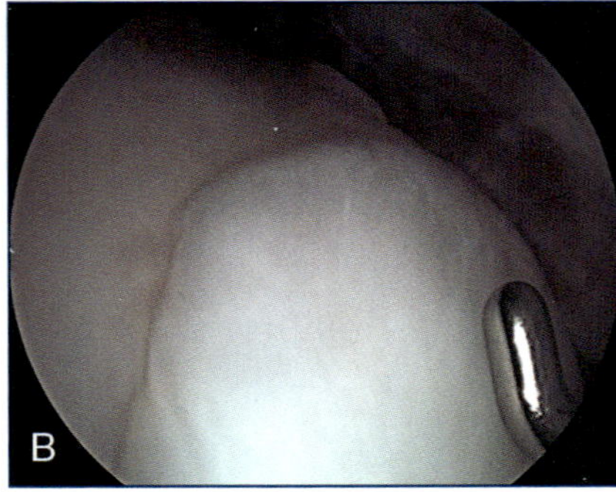

Figure 1 Periosteal hypertrophy after ACI. **A,** Sagittal T2-weighted fast spin-echo, fat-suppressed, proton density MRI shows a hypertrophic ACI graft of the medial femoral condyle. Note the artifact from the high tibial osteotomy hardware. **B,** Arthroscopic image demonstrates the hypertrophic graft. Note the prominent, bulging tissue that is raised several millimeters above the level of the surrounding cartilage.

Complication

Nine months postoperatively, the patient noticed increasing popping and clicking, but no locking of the joint. The symptoms started insidiously and there was no significant trauma. Physical examination demonstrated reproducible clicking at approximately 30° of flexion on flexion-extension of the knee.

Treatment

Nonsurgical treatment of the complication with activity modification was tried for more than 3 months, but the symptoms persisted. The patient underwent arthroscopy with débridement of a hypertrophic periosteal patch.

Outcome

The patient recovered uneventfully and was functioning well without symptoms more than 2 years after his original surgery. Treatment for the complication occurred 1 year after the index procedure with 1 year additional follow-up time after the débridement.

Discussion

Periosteal hypertrophy, which is associated with the use of a periosteal patch to cover the defect, is a common problem after ACI. It occurs in 20% to 50% of patients,[3,4] and its incidence is highest after patellar ACI.[2] Since the introduction of collagen membranes to replace periosteum in Europe, the incidence of hypertrophy has dropped to almost 0%.[5]

Recognizing the Problem

Patients with periosteal hypertrophy frequently present with increasing mechanical symptoms between 6 and 12 months after ACI. An increase in activity level may precede the symptoms. Popping or clicking occasionally can be reproduced at certain flexion angles. Pain, swelling, and effusion can occur, but they are not always present.

Treating the Problem

Attempts should be made to treat symptoms nonsurgically, with a period of activity modification including weight-bearing restrictions with crutches and decreased or paused physical therapy, and short-term anti-inflammatory medication (1 to 2 weeks). If symptoms do not improve, further treatment depends on the level of symptoms. If the symptoms are tolerable, no intervention is necessary; however, if symptoms are disabling, then an MRI (**Figure 1,** *A*) should be obtained to assess the graft and distinguish between hypertrophy and graft failure due to delamination.

If hypertrophy is the cause of intolerable symptoms, arthroscopic débridement can provide predictable relief. Adhesions in the anterior interval are common after arthrotomy and can complicate atraumatic insertion of the arthroscope. A hemostat clamp

© 2011 American Academy of Orthopaedic Surgeons

or similar instrument helps spread through the fat pad and capsule, followed by a switching stick and finally the arthroscopic cannula. Alternatively, the arthroscope can be introduced through an accessory superolateral portal.

If the graft is found to be prominent by several millimeters, usually due to hypertrophy of the periosteal patch, it can be carefully debulked to the level of the surrounding cartilage (**Figure 1,** *B*). This should be performed with a shaver, not an electrothermal device, and ideally should be limited to the fibrous cap of the hypertrophied periosteal membrane without removing any regenerated cartilage tissue.

Preventing the Problem

Periosteal hypertrophy can be virtually eliminated by the use of a resorbable collagen membrane in place of periosteum. Although such membranes have been used in Europe for almost 10 years, none are currently approved by the US Food and Drug Administration for ACI in the United States. Their use remains off-label but is becoming increasingly popular with American surgeons.[6]

Case 2: Graft Delamination

History

A 25-year-old man presented with varus alignment of the lower extremity and a large chondral defect of the medial femoral condyle. He was treated with ACI for an 8-cm^2 defect with concurrent high tibial osteotomy and recovered uneventfully.

Complication

Six months after the procedure, the patient sustained a twisting injury to his knee, with a sudden increase in pain and mechanical symptoms. These symptoms failed to respond to activity restrictions, partial weight bearing on crutches, and anti-inflammatory therapy for 2 weeks. The patient previously had recovered well from his index surgery and had been ambulating without pain before this episode. Examination demonstrated mild swelling and a small effusion and range of motion from full extension to 140° of flexion with good patellar mobility. Radiographs demonstrated a healed high tibial osteotomy and preserved joint spaces throughout. MRI showed partial delamination of the posterior aspect of the graft (**Figure 2,** *A*).

Treatment

The patient underwent arthroscopy to evaluate the graft, which demonstrated delamination of otherwise healthy-appearing repair tissue. The tissue was débrided and the residual defect, which measured 3 cm^2, was microfractured.

Outcome

The patient recovered uneventfully and was functioning well 2 years after the débridement and microfracture.

Discussion

Graft delamination with ACI is rare (<5%), but when it does occur, the patient usually presents within the first 2 years after implantation.[2] Usually, healthy-appearing repair tissue forms and the patient becomes less symptomatic or asymptomatic. Then, either with or without specific trauma, the patient experiences a sharp increase in pain, often with mechanical symptoms such as clicking, popping, or even locking of the knee.

Recognizing the Problem

Temporary setbacks are common after ACI, but they usually respond to symptomatic treatment with activity restriction and anti-inflammatory therapy. If symptoms fail to respond to appropriate therapy, MRI should be considered, ideally with contrast material, to increase sensitivity for delamination. With MRI evidence or suspicion for delamination, arthroscopy should be considered to evaluate the graft. Treatment options should be discussed with the patient, including microfracture or osteochondral autograft transfer for partial delamination, and removal of the graft if a larger portion or the entire graft is affected.

Treating the Problem

The entire joint should be carefully evaluated, in particular all graft sites. A delaminated graft can appear innocuous (**Figure 2,** *B*) until probed (**Figure 2,** *C*). All detached tissue should be removed back to a stable rim[2-4] (**Figure 2,** *D*). Depending on the size of the

© 2011 American Academy of Orthopaedic Surgeons

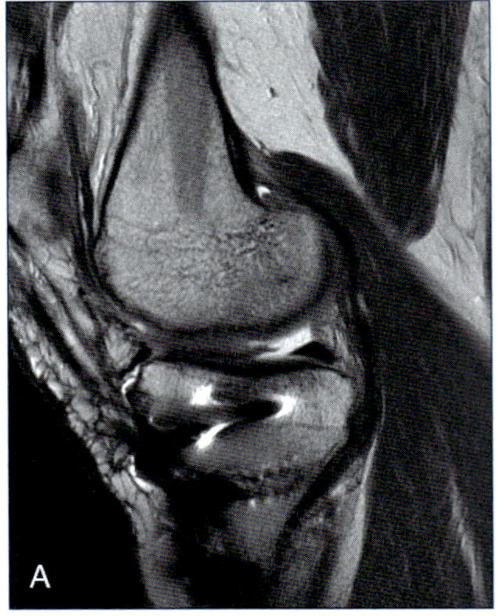

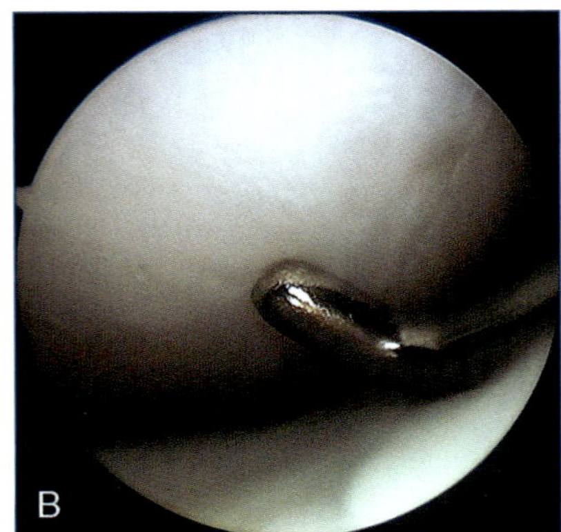

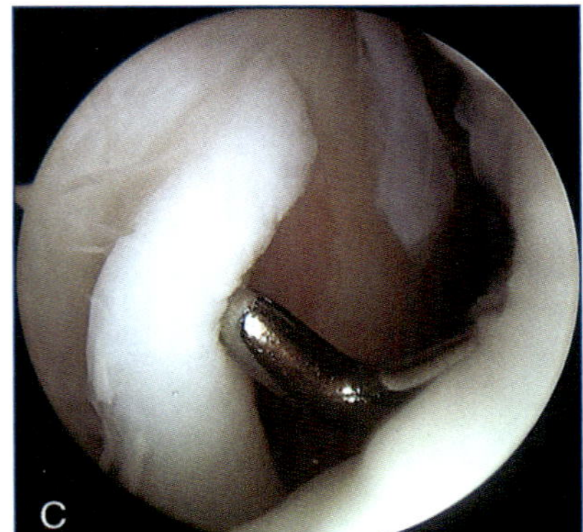

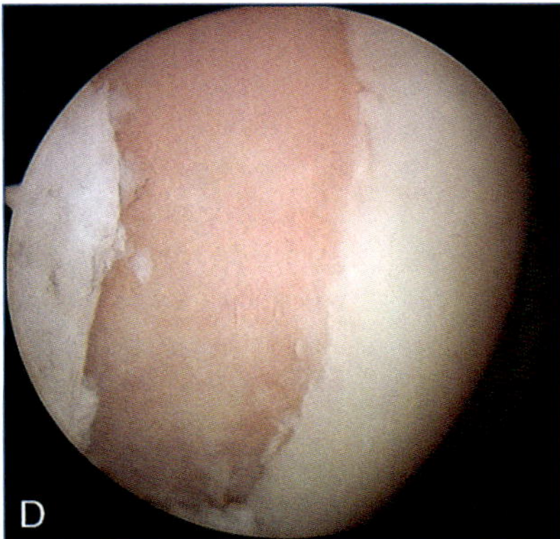

Figure 2 Graft delamination after ACI. **A,** Sagittal T1-weighted fast spin-echo, proton density MRI with indirect gadolinium enhancement demonstrates partial delamination of the posterior aspect of an ACI graft in the medial femoral condyle. **B,** Arthroscopic view shows the graft apparently intact with good fill and integration. **C,** Arthroscopic view demonstrates instability and delamination of otherwise healthy-appearing graft tissue upon probing. **D,** Arthroscopic view of the graft site after débridement of all unstable tissue.

resulting defect, an appropriate cartilage repair method should be chosen to address the lesion. Partial delamination results in lesions smaller than the originally treated defect, and these can be amenable to microfracture or osteochondral autograft transfer at the time of arthroscopic evaluation. Therefore, the potential for these procedures and their respective recovery times should always be discussed with the patient whenever a diagnostic arthroscopy is performed to evaluate symptoms after ACI.

If the entire graft has delaminated, revision surgery with repeat ACI, osteochondral allograft, or prosthetic replacement is indicated, depending on the reason for failure. If the subchondral bone is intact and good cartilage had formed that subsequently delaminated, revision with ACI is preferable. If the subchondral bone is overly abnormal (cysts or significant sclerosis) or the regenerated tissue mainly consists of fibrotic scar, then osteochondral allograft transplantation should be considered. If the remaining joint demonstrates significant arthritic changes at this point (progression of disease), then prosthetic replacement can be considered.

Preventing the Problem

The repair tissue after ACI remains vulnerable to injury, particularly from shear forces, for 12 to 18 months. Patients should be cautioned to adhere to the rehabilitation protocol with slow progression and avoidance of any pivoting, twisting, or high-impact activities for at least 12 months.

© 2011 American Academy of Orthopaedic Surgeons

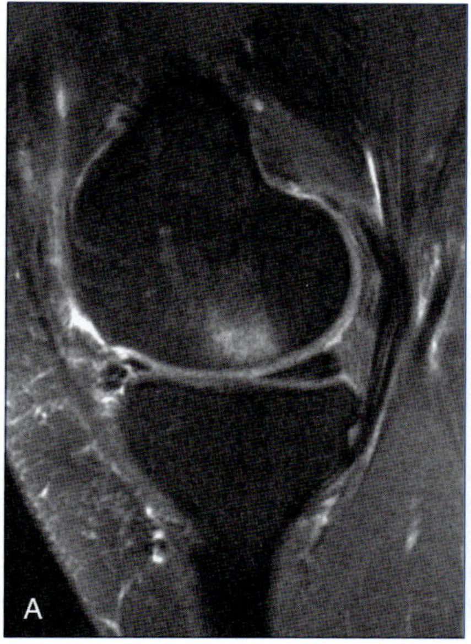

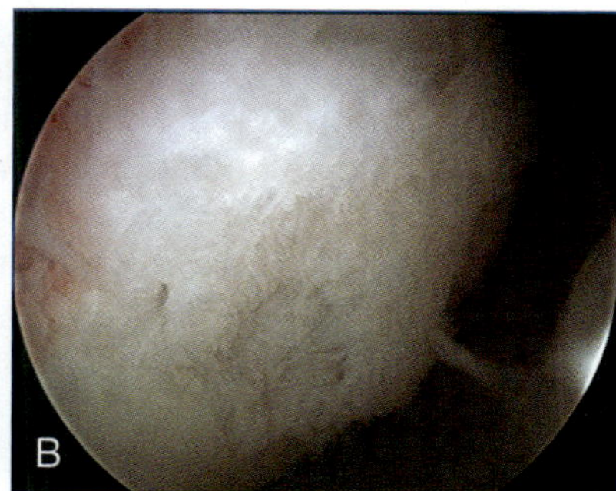

Figure 3 Biologic failure after ACI. **A,** Sagittal T2-weighted MRI shows persistent bone marrow edema underlying an ACI graft site on the medial femoral condyle 18 months after implantation. The graft site demonstrates good fill with reparative tissue. **B,** Arthroscopic view shows fibrous scar instead of hyaline-like repair tissue.

Case 3: Biologic Failure

History

A 22-year-old woman presented with persistent medial joint-line pain due to a 5-cm² chondral defect of the medial femoral condyle. Because alignment was normal, the patient was treated with ACI alone. Her postoperative course was remarkable for prolonged swelling and persistent pain with weight-bearing activities.

Complication and Treatment

At 12 months, the patient's symptoms failed to improve, even with activity modification and anti-inflammatory therapy. She remarked that the pain was similar to her preoperative symptoms. Examination demonstrated mild swelling and a small effusion, range of motion from near-full extension to 130° of flexion, and mild tenderness to palpation of the medial femoral condyle and joint line. Radiographs demonstrated well-preserved joint spaces. MRI demonstrated good coverage of the repair site with tissue and no delamination but persistent subchondral bone marrow edema (**Figure 3,** *A*). The patient underwent arthroscopy, which demonstrated fibrous scar tissue at the repair site (**Figure 3,** *B*).

Outcome

The patient was treated with repeat cartilage biopsy and revision ACI. She was doing well 3 years postoperatively.

Discussion

Biologic failure of the implant can occur as a result of inadequate growth with underfill of the defect or formation of a fibrous, rather than hyaline, tissue. In both instances, the resultant tissue inadequately protects the underlying subchondral bone, leading to incomplete pain relief. Depending on the degree and duration of symptoms, revision surgery is indicated.

Recognizing the Problem

With persistent symptoms unresponsive to appropriate nonsurgical management and MRI evidence of graft abnormality or persistent (longer than 12 months) subchondral bone marrow edema, arthroscopic evaluation is recommended to evaluate the graft.

Treating the Problem

Diagnostic arthroscopy is performed to evaluate the graft sites. Consent should be obtained from patients for the possibility of cartilage repair with microfracture or osteochondral autograft in case of partial graft failure.

© 2011 American Academy of Orthopaedic Surgeons

The graft is carefully evaluated and probed to determine stability and integration. Any residual tissue from the periosteal or collagen patch can be gently and carefully débrided with the shaver to expose the graft itself. Occasionally, the graft is found to be well integrated and of good tissue quality; in this case, continued nonsurgical treatment with activity modification, unloader bracing, and anti-inflammatory drugs should be pursued. In some of these patients, the graft will continue on to late delamination.

Occasionally, the regenerative tissue is found on superficial débridement to consist of fibrous scar (**Figure 3,** *B*) rather than hyaline-like cartilage. In this case, depending on the size of the lesion affected, revision surgery should be performed with either repeat ACI or osteochondral allograft.

Preventing the Problem

Few data are available on the prevention of biologic graft failure (ie, inadequate fill or formation of a fibrous scar). Meticulous surgical technique is important to provide a dry surgical bed without significant bleeding from the subchondral plate, which could dilute the end-differentiated chondrocytes with marrow cells, producing a more fibrous repair tissue. Furthermore, bleeding or inadequate waterproofing of the suture line can lead to leakage of chondrocytes from the defect, potentially compromising the formation of a robust repair tissue.

Case 4: Arthrofibrosis

History

A 32-year-old man on chronic pain medication was treated with ACI and tibial tubercle osteotomy for a 6-cm^2 central trochlear defect. The postoperative course was remarkable for significant pain control issues that complicated use of a continuous passive motion machine and physical therapy for range-of-motion exercises.

Complication and Treatment

Ten weeks after ACI, the patient had transitioned to full weight bearing as instructed but was having difficulty regaining a normal gait because of restricted range of motion in the knee. According to the physical therapy report, the patient had been unable to improve the range of motion in the last 4 weeks despite a stretching regimen. Examination showed diffuse soft-tissue swelling, no effusion, and moderate quadriceps atrophy. The patient had near-full extension but limited flexion to 50° (**Figure 4,** *A*), with very limited patellar mobility. Radiographs demonstrated a healing tibial tubercle osteotomy.

Surgical intervention for lysis of adhesions was recommended at this point because of the lack of progress for 4 weeks, with very limited motion and patellar mobility. Open versus arthroscopic lysis of adhesions was discussed with the patient. The plan was to proceed with an arthroscopic intervention because the patient had a 50° arc of motion and was only 10 weeks out from the index procedure. Dense scar tissue was encountered in both gutters, the anterior interval, and the suprapatellar pouch. The fat pad was adherent to the trochlear graft. The patient was treated with an arthroscopic lysis of adhesions as described below.

Outcome

The patient regained 135° of flexion and was weaned off pain medications.

Discussion

Arthrofibrosis is seen in 5% to 10% of patients after ACI and should be treated aggressively and early. Because the graft is friable during the first 6 to 12 weeks after surgery, there are limits to stretching by physical therapy, both manually and with progressive splinting. Closed manipulation has no role after ACI because of frequent adhesion formation between capsule and grafts, with the potential for graft avulsion with forced motion.

Recognizing the Problem

Generally, knees that fail to progress beyond 70° of flexion by 6 weeks will not reach normal motion even with extended physical therapy and should be considered for lysis of adhesions.

Treating the Problem

Aggressive stretching might improve motion but risks damage to what is, at 12 weeks after surgery, still considered an immature graft. Delaying surgical intervention allows the scar tissue to mature further, obliterating tissue planes and complicating lysis of adhesions.

© 2011 American Academy of Orthopaedic Surgeons

Both open and arthroscopic lysis of adhesions should always be discussed with the patient, with a preference for arthroscopy because of its lower morbidity. Generally, patients with milder forms of arthrofibrosis and a motion arc of 45° or more can be treated arthroscopically, especially when surgery was performed recently (within 3 months). Cases of more severe arthrofibrosis with near ankylosis (<20° to 30° arc of motion), significant postoperative patella infera, and longer history of decreased motion should be considered for open lysis of adhesions and, potentially, proximalization of the tibial tubercle.

Arthroscopic Lysis of Adhesions

Arthroscopic lysis of adhesions is best performed using a tourniquet to improve visualization. The knee is injected with saline to insufflate the joint and facilitate portal placement. A superolateral portal is created; a switching stick is placed into the suprapatellar pouch and exchanged for the arthroscope. Next, an inferolateral portal is created under direct visualization. Frequently, the medial and lateral patellar retinaculae are contracted, making it impossible to move instruments or the arthroscope between the patella and the trochlea. Therefore, a lateral retinacular release is performed, connecting the two portal sites. This release can be facilitated first by creating a plane between the subcutaneous tissues and the capsule, which is then divided with the electrothermal device. The lateral gutter is then freed of adhesions (**Figure 4,** *B*), which usually allows instruments to pass freely through the patellofemoral joint. Next, the graft sites are inspected and any adhesions are carefully removed with the shaver (**Figure 4,** *C*). At this point, the knee can be flexed, and a medial portal is created under direct visualization. An anterior interval release is performed, dividing adhesions that commonly connect the inferior pole of the patella with the intermeniscal ligament or anterior cruciate ligament. This release connects the inferomedial and inferolateral portals, staying anterior to the intermeniscal ligament and cutting distally along the anterior surface of the proximal tibia toward the tibial tubercle. It is critical to protect the patellar tendon, which is at risk during this part of the procedure. Once the scar tissue has been divided along the intermeniscal ligament, it can be removed with an aggressive shaver until the Hoffa fat pad is visualized. If patellar mobility is still limited, a medial retinacular release should be performed. Although the corresponding capsular release extends laterally to the vastus lateralis tendon close to the superior pole of the patella, I prefer to stop at the mid level of the patella for the medial capsular release to decrease the risk of creating iatrogenic patellar instability. Finally, the suprapatellar pouch is inspected and any adhesions (**Figure 4,** *D*) are released with the electrothermal device, staying close to the femur to avoid injury to the quadriceps tendon. My colleagues and I prefer to perform this last because fluid extravasation into the thigh occurs once the adhesions have been released in this area. Last, the knee is gently manipulated to assess motion and to break up any remaining adhesions (**Figure 4,** *E*). I prefer using a suction drain, which the patient removes at home on postoperative day 1 or 2; these patients are treated prophylactically with oral antibiotics until the drain has been removed. Continuous passive motion is started the next day, progressing quickly to 110° of flexion. Physical therapy for range-of-motion stretching and patellar mobilization is critical and usually starts within a few days after surgery to preserve motion (**Figure 4,** *F*).

Open Lysis of Adhesions

The previous skin incision usually can be used for open lysis of adhesions. Full-thickness fasciocutaneous flaps are raised medially and laterally, extending from the level of the tibial tubercle to the proximal pole of the patella. Adhesions between the subcutaneous tissues and the quadriceps tendon should be released. The medial and lateral borders of the patellar tendon are dissected free, and medial and lateral subvastus approaches are used. The vastus medialis and lateralis are followed proximally and posteriorly to the intermuscular septum, from which they are carefully elevated, being mindful of perforating blood vessels. The synovial reflection of the suprapatellar pouch is frequently obliterated with dense scar tissue. A tissue plane is developed between the femur and the undersurface of the quadriceps tendon and muscle just proximal to this scar tissue, which is then sharply divided. Any adhesions between the quadriceps and femur are now released with an elevator, moving proximally along the femur. Finally, a plane between the patellar tendon and anterior proximal tibia is developed, starting at the tibial tubercle insertion of the patellar tendon. This plane is followed proximal-

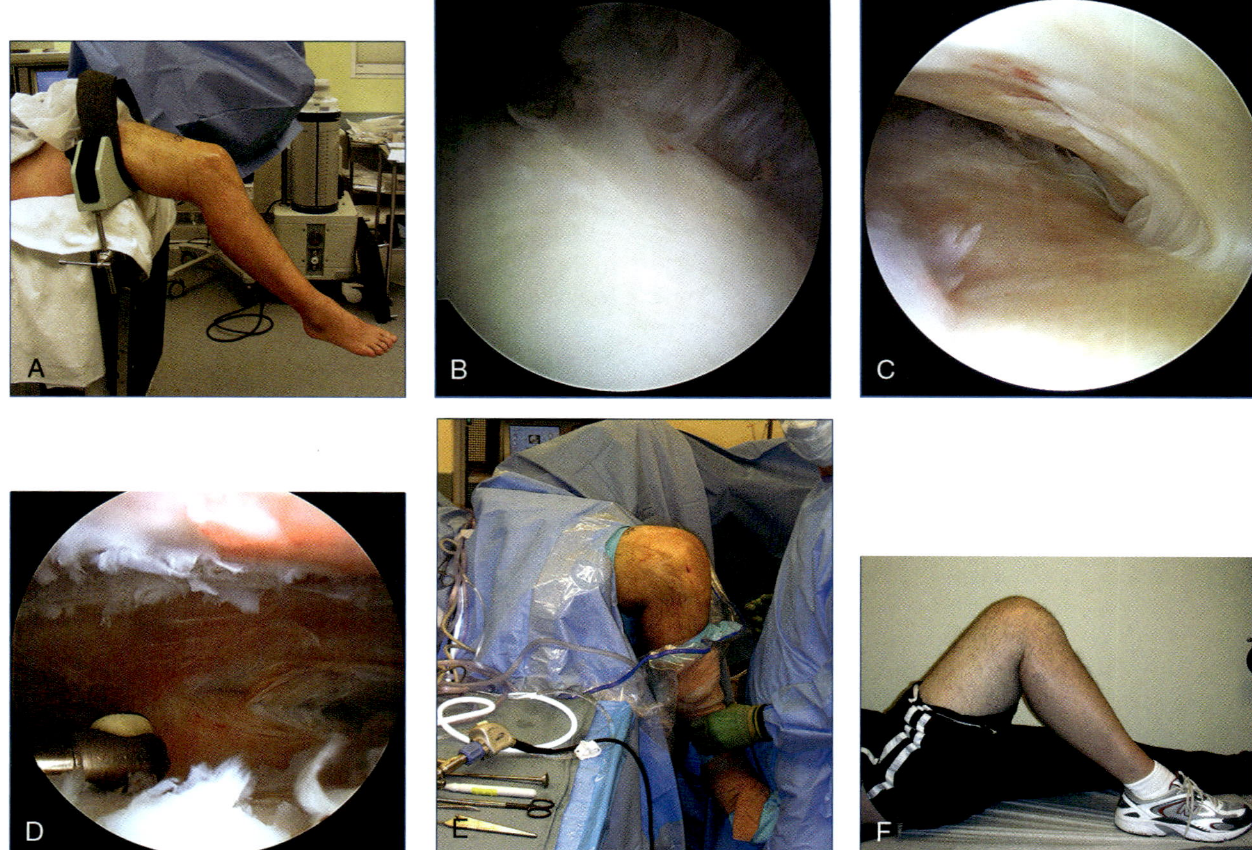

Figure 4 Arthrofibrosis after ACI. **A,** Preoperative photograph demonstrates limited flexion. **B** through **D** are arthroscopic views obtained with the knee in extension. **B,** View through a superomedial portal shows the lateral gutter obliterated by adhesions (right is proximal; left is distal). **C,** View through a superolateral portal shows an adhesion between the fat pad and a trochlear ACI graft (right is distal; left is proximal). **D,** View through an inferolateral portal shows adhesions in the suprapatellar pouch. **E,** Photograph shows the knee being gently manipulated to assess motion and to break up any remaining adhesions. **F,** Postoperative clinical photograph of the knee shows improved flexion.

ly along the anterior tibia, dividing the fat pad just anterior to the intermeniscal ligament. Densely fibrosed tissue should be excised, but ideally the fat pad should not be completely removed.

Case 5: Setbacks During Rehabilitation

History

A 38-year-old woman presented with a large full-thickness chondral defect of the central trochlea and was treated with ACI. Early recovery was uneventful, with restoration of near-normal motion.

Complication and Treatment

Four months after surgery, the patient noticed pain and swelling above her baseline for more than 1 week. She denied any traumatic event, fevers, or chills. On discussion of her recent activities, she reported returning recently from vacation where she had visited an amusement park with her children and ambulated much more than usual. Examination showed soft-tissue swelling, a large effusion, and

© 2011 American Academy of Orthopaedic Surgeons

warmth, but no erythema of the knee joint. Motion was unchanged.

She was placed back on crutches for 2 weeks with partial weight bearing and cryotherapy, physical therapy for edema control, and nonsteroidal anti-inflammatory drugs for 1 week.

Outcome

The flare-up resolved within 2 weeks. The patient was functioning well 2 years after ACI.

Discussion

Rehabilitation after ACI is prolonged. Ideally, the mechanical loads placed on the joint should steadily and slowly increase with the maturation of the graft to avoid overloading the graft and underlying subchondral bone.

Recognizing the Problem

Symptoms above the established baseline that last for more than 1 week should be investigated and addressed.

Treating the Problem

Patients should be carefully questioned on their recent activity levels. Any increased activity level can lead to large effusions, a sense of stiffness, and pain. A distinct traumatic incident with subsequent symptoms should be evaluated with MRI; otherwise, a trial of nonsurgical management should be attempted first. Depending on the level of symptoms, patients should curtail their activities, or even go back on crutches with protected weight bearing for up to 2 weeks. Elevation and cryotherapy are important components as well. Oral anti-inflammatory drugs should be used, but my preference is to limit this to less than 2 weeks because of the potential negative effects on cartilage healing. If no improvement occurs after 2 to 3 weeks, gadolinium-enhanced MRI is indicated to rule out graft delamination.

Preventing the Problem

The repair tissue after ACI remains soft for 6 to 9 months and is unable to protect the subchondral bone from sudden increases in activity levels; inflammation and effusion can develop. Slow increases in activity levels, both during daily chores and sports, can help avoid flare-ups.

Summary

ACI is a challenging procedure for the surgeon, with regard to indications and technique, and for the patient, who undergoes a prolonged recovery time of 12 to 18 months. Strict adherence to surgical technique and postoperative rehabilitation guidelines minimizes the risk of complications and leads to successful outcomes in more than 80% of patients.

References

1. Brittberg M, Lindahl A, Nilsson A, Ohlsson C, Isaksson O, Peterson L: Treatment of deep cartilage defects in the knee with autologous chondrocyte transplantation. *N Engl J Med* 1994;331(14):889-895.
2. Niemeyer P, Pestka JM, Kreuz PC, et al: Characteristic complications after autologous chondrocyte implantation for cartilage defects of the knee joint. *Am J Sports Med* 2008;36(11):2091-2099.
3. Kreuz PC, Steinwachs M, Erggelet C, et al: Classification of graft hypertrophy after autologous chondrocyte implantation of full-thickness chondral defects in the knee. *Osteoarthritis Cartilage* 2007;15(12):1339-1347.
4. Minas T, Gomoll AH, Solhpour S, Rosenberger R, Probst C, Bryant T: Autologous chondrocyte implantation for joint preservation in patients with early osteoarthritis. *Clin Orthop Relat Res* 2010;468(1): 147-157.
5. Gooding CR, Bartlett W, Bentley G, Skinner JA, Carrington R, Flanagan A: A prospective, randomised study comparing two techniques of autologous chondrocyte implantation for osteochondral defects in the knee: Periosteum covered versus type I/III collagen covered. *Knee* 2006;13(3):203-210.
6. Gomoll AH, Probst C, Farr J, Cole BJ, Minas T: Use of a type I/III bilayer collagen membrane decreases reoperation rates for symptomatic hypertrophy after autologous chondrocyte implantation. *Am J Sports Med* 2009;37(Suppl 1):20S-23S.

© 2011 American Academy of Orthopaedic Surgeons

Chapter 5

High Tibial Osteotomy/ Distal Femoral Osteotomy

Annunziato Amendola, MD
Davide Edoardo Bonasia, MD

Introduction

High tibial osteotomy (HTO) and distal femoral osteotomy (DFO) are reliable procedures to treat medial and lateral arthrosis of the knee, respectively. Even though outcomes deteriorate with time, careful patient selection and precise surgical technique provide good to excellent long-term results. Recent studies have shown a 54% to 90% survivorship of HTO at 15 to 20 years.[1-3] Currently, the most common indication for HTO/DFO is isolated unicompartmental arthrosis of the knee, usually in patients too young to undergo knee arthroplasty.

We strongly believe that alignment critically influences the outcome of every cartilage resurfacing procedure. A cartilage salvage/repair procedure is more likely to fail if performed in an overloaded compartment. Alignment correction is essential to achieve durable results. Abrasion arthroplasty, microfracture, autologous chondrocyte implantation, and meniscal transplantation all have been described in association with HTO. The results are considered controversial because of the lack of randomized controlled trials comparing resurfacing procedures performed alone and in association with osteotomy in malaligned knees.[4] We believe that unloading a damaged compartment of the knee with osteotomy is essential, both to prevent further damage and to assist healing of any associated cartilage repair procedure. Malalignment can be both cause and consequence of chondral damage and has to be corrected for cartilage repair to be successful.

Nevertheless, osteotomy is an invasive procedure and is associated with complications including fracture, nonunion, infection, modified patellar height, compartment syndrome, peroneal nerve palsy, and thromboembolism.

Dr. Amendola or a member of his immediate family serves as a board member, owner, officer, or committee member of the American Orthopaedic Society for Sports Medicine and the Iowa Donor Network; has received royalties from Arthrex; serves as a paid consultant to or is an employee of Arthrex and Arthrosurface; and owns stock or stock options in Arthrosurface. Neither Dr. Bonasia nor any immediate family member has received anything of value from or owns stock in a commercial company or institution related directly or indirectly to the subject of this chapter.

© 2011 American Academy of Orthopaedic Surgeons

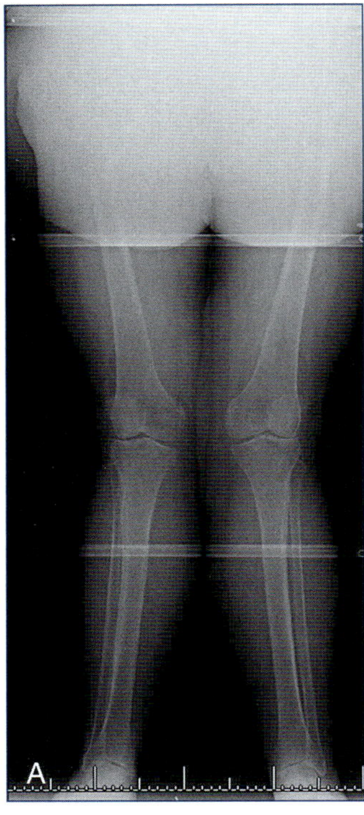

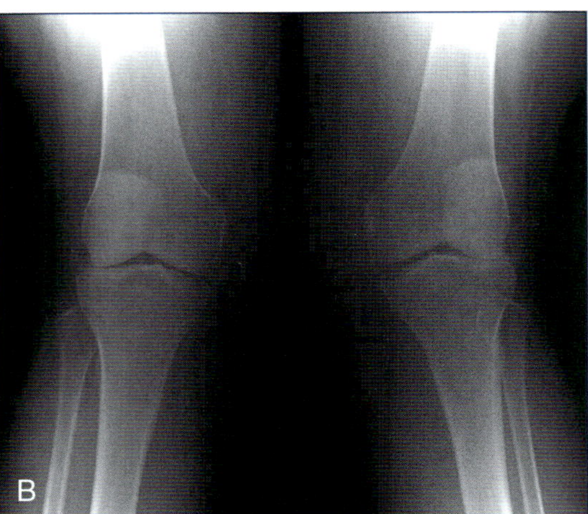

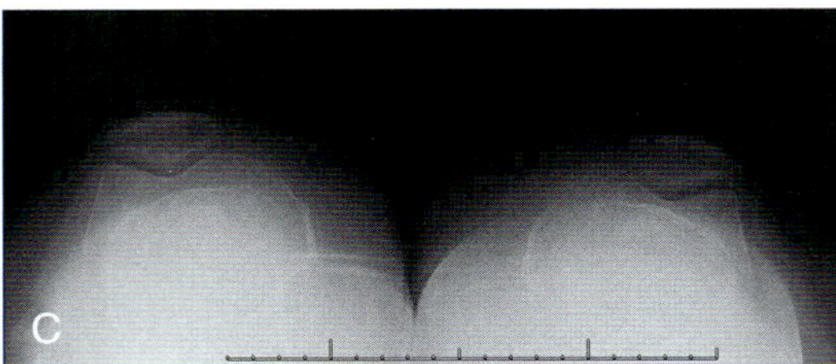

Figure 1 Preoperative images of the 47-year-old woman described in case 1. **A,** AP long-leg weight-bearing radiograph shows valgus alignment of both limbs. **B,** AP weight-bearing radiograph shows lateral compartment arthrosis of both knees. **C,** Merchant view shows preserved patellofemoral compartments.

Case 1: Delayed Union and Loss of Correction

History

A 47-year-old woman presented with constant activity-related left knee pain. On physical examination, the patient was slightly overweight, with valgus alignment of both knees. Range of motion of the left knee was 0° to 125°, with pain at maximal degrees of flexion. The pain was mainly lateral. The medial and patellofemoral compartments were normal. Preoperative radiographs confirmed bilateral valgus malalignment and lateral unicompartmental arthritis (**Figure 1**). The patient underwent a lateral opening wedge DFO without intraoperative complications (**Figure 2**).

Current Problem and Management

At 6- and 12-week follow-up, delayed union and loss of correction were evident (**Figure 3**). Revision surgery was not required. The rehabilitation protocol was delayed. Partial weight bearing was allowed at 3 months after surgery and full weight bearing at 4 months.

Outcome

At 6-month follow-up, the patient was doing well and the osteotomy had healed without any further loss of correction (**Figure 4**). Pain during daily activities was noticeably reduced, and the range of motion was 0° to 120°.

Discussion

Recognizing the Problem

Delayed union with or without loss of correction is a common complication in HTO and DFO. The incidence of delayed union is 6.6% in medial opening wedge osteotomy and 8.5% in lateral closing wedge osteotomy.[5]

Managing the Problem

Early recognition of delayed healing and loss of correction is achieved with thorough follow-up, from immediately after surgery through complete healing

© 2011 American Academy of Orthopaedic Surgeons

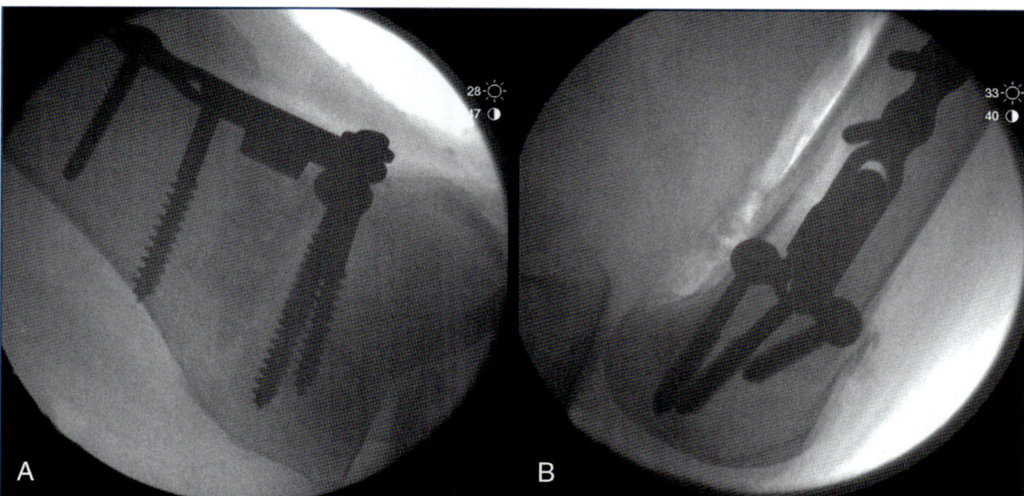

Figure 2 Intraoperative images of the same patient shown in Figure 1 obtained during a lateral opening wedge DFO of the left knee. AP (**A**) and lateral (**B**) fluoroscopic images show no apparent complications.

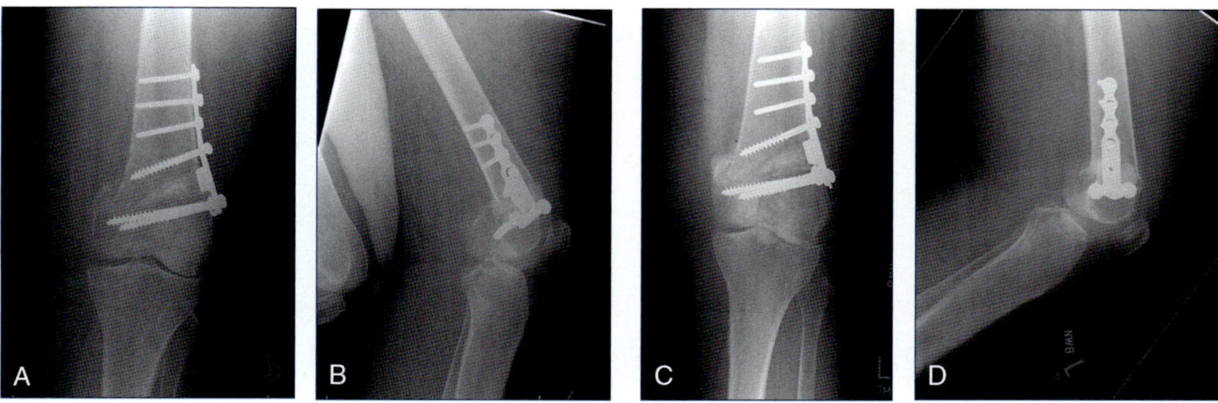

Figure 3 Postoperative images of the same patient shown in Figure 1. AP (**A**) and lateral (**B**) views obtained at 6 weeks and AP (**C**) and lateral (**D**) views obtained at 12 weeks show delayed union and loss of correction.

of the osteotomy. Short radiographs are obtained 6 and 12 weeks postoperatively to monitor maintenance of correction and healing, and long-leg films are obtained 6 months postoperatively to assess the alignment achieved.[6]

If delayed union or an unstable construct that may lead to delayed union is recognized postoperatively, a cautious rehabilitation protocol—one that prolongs the non–weight-bearing phase until radiographic evidence of osteotomy healing is seen—should be considered. In most cases, this management is successful in avoiding loss of correction and nonunion. If only slight loss of correction occurs (3° to 5°), the patient's symptoms should guide the decision to consider revision. If a more severe loss of correction is recognized, revision is indicated, with realignment and alternate fixation using a different device.

Preventing the Problem

Careful patient selection is the first step in preventing delayed union. Smokers have a higher risk of delayed union and nonunion.[7] For this reason, it is mandatory to emphasize the importance of quitting smoking with a compliant patient or to plan a different sur-

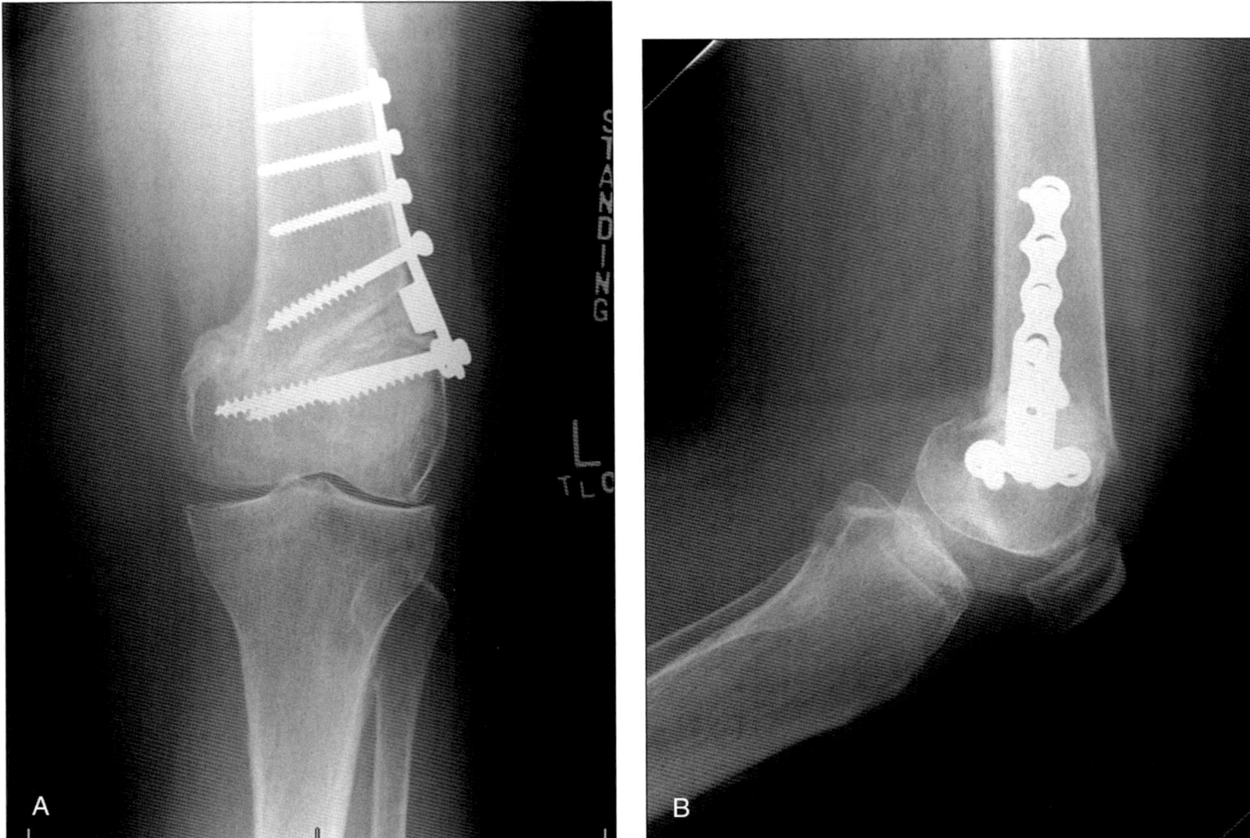

Figure 4 Postoperative images of the same patient shown in Figure 1 obtained at 6-month follow-up. AP (**A**) and lateral (**B**) views show complete healing and no further loss of correction.

gery with a noncompliant patient (eg, closing wedge osteotomy or unicompartmental knee arthroplasty, when indicated).

Opening wedge osteotomy creates a situation in which biologic healing of the opening has to occur and the osteotomy has to consolidate for a successful outcome. The method used to fill the osseous gap is considered an important factor in influencing the osteotomy healing rate, even though no evidence has been reported in the literature.[7] Many techniques have been used, including bone grafts (autograft or allograft) and synthetic bone substitutes (hydroxyapatite, β-tricalcium phosphate, or a combination of both; or bone cement).[4] Platelet-rich plasma, growth factors, and bone marrow stromal cells are being investigated to augment grafting techniques.[8] Autograft bone generally is considered to be the gold standard because of its osteoconductive, osteoinductive, and osteogenic properties.[9-11] The drawbacks of autograft include increased surgical time and donor-site morbidity. Therefore, autologous iliac crest bone graft is recommended in high-risk situations (eg, obese patient, smoker, opening angle >10°, revision procedures).[7] On the other hand, allografts have reduced osteoinductive properties and involve the risk of disease transmission. Synthetic bone substitutes are used in an attempt to reduce the risks associated with bone grafting. These materials have good biologic degradability, but a

© 2011 American Academy of Orthopaedic Surgeons

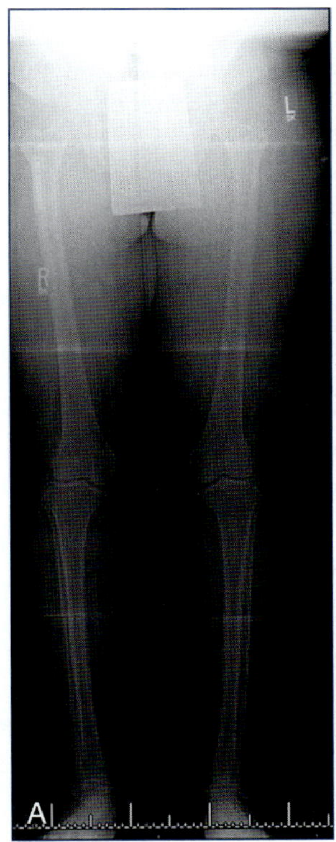

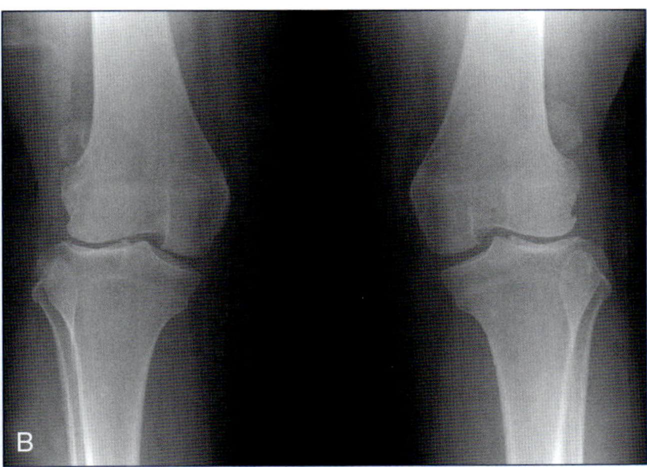

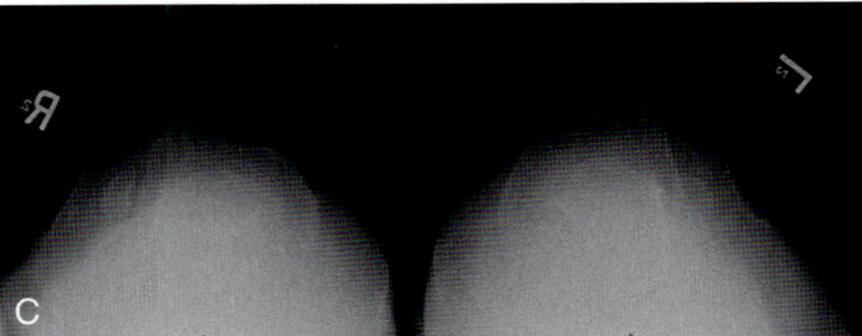

Figure 5 Preoperative images of the 41-year-old woman described in case 2. AP long-leg weight-bearing (**A**), AP (**B**), and Merchant (**C**) radiographs show bilateral severe varus tibial malalignment, moderate valgus femoral malalignment, and chronic patellar dislocation.

major issue is the low resistance of macroporous ceramics against compressive loads.[7] The use of bone cement as a spacer has been described[12] but is not widespread because of its lack of integration and desorption.[7] Controversy still exists regarding the most reliable augmentation technique.

Another factor that may affect healing and cause loss of correction is an aggressive rehabilitation protocol. A standard postoperative regimen, which is somewhat more restricted than that for the closing wedge procedure, should be followed after opening wedge osteotomies.[6] For the first 6 weeks, the knee is placed in a range-of-motion brace set at 0° to 90°, and the patient is encouraged to achieve this range, particularly full extension. During this period, the patient continues crutch-assisted toe-touch weight bearing. From 6 to 12 weeks postoperatively, the brace is discontinued and weight bearing is progressed gradually to full weight bearing. From 3 to 6 months postoperatively, the patient is encouraged to increase activities as tolerated.[6]

Case 2: Medial/Lateral Hinge Disruption and Nonunion

History

A 41-year-old woman presented with severe bilateral knee pain. She has been previously diagnosed with congenital bilateral patellar dislocation. On physical examination, the patient was overweight, with a slight varus alignment of both knees. Both patellae were hypoplastic and laterally dislocated. Range of motion was 0° to 110° in both knees. The pain was mainly located in the medial compartment of the knee. Preoperative radiographs confirmed severe varus tibial malalignment, moderate valgus femoral malalignment, and patellar dislocation (**Figure 5**).

The patient underwent surgery on the left knee, consisting of opening wedge HTO in conjunction with opening wedge DFO, patellectomy, and extensor mechanism distal realignment tibial tubercle osteotomy (TTO). Intraoperatively, both the femoral

© 2011 American Academy of Orthopaedic Surgeons

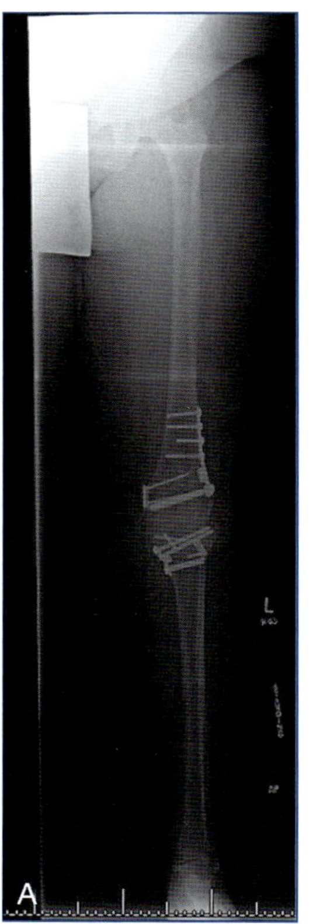

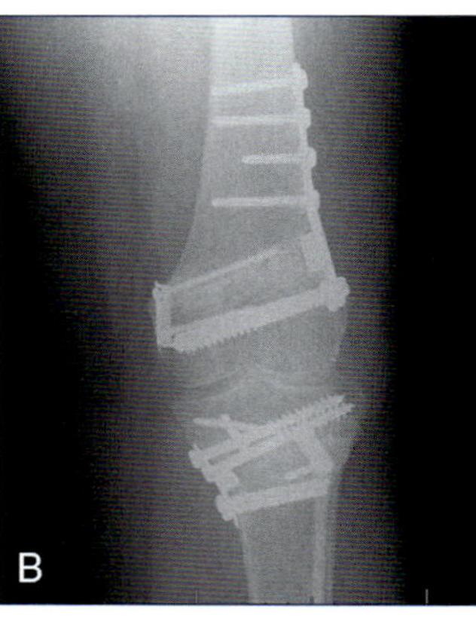

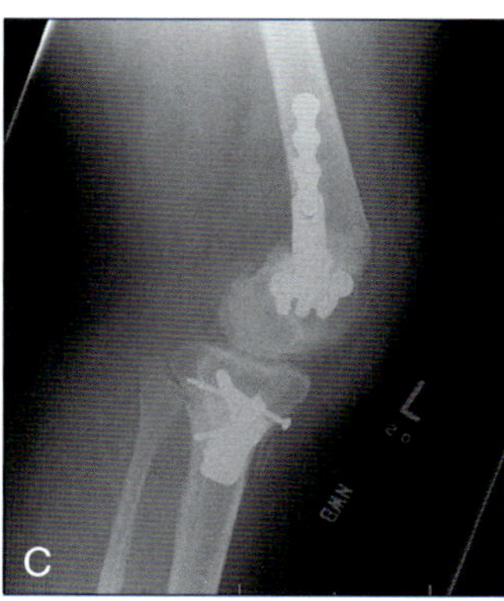

Figure 6 Images of the same patient shown in Figure 5 obtained 6 months after undergoing opening wedge HTO and DFO, patellectomy, and extensor mechanism distal realignment of the left knee. AP long-leg weight-bearing (**A**), AP (**B**), and lateral (**C**) radiographs show complete healing of the osteotomies. On both the femoral and the tibial side, a two-hole plate was added to restore the medial and lateral hinges because they were disrupted intraoperatively.

medial hinge and lateral tibial hinge failed because of the poor bone quality and the great amount of correction needed. Additional two-hole plates were used to restore hinge stability. At 6-month follow-up, healing was evident at both osteotomy sites, the pain was significantly improved, and the patient was happy with the outcome (**Figure 6**). One year after the first surgery, the patient returned for the same procedure on the contralateral (right) knee. On the femoral side, the medial hinge failed intraoperatively and was stabilized with an additional two-hole plate. The lateral HTO hinge showed no disruption on fluoroscopy. At immediate postoperative follow-up, a fracture line was seen on radiographs that directed distally from the tibial osteotomy site (**Figure 7**, *A* and *B*). At 6-week follow-up, radiographic evidence was encouraging. No loss of correction or hardware breakage was seen (**Figure 7**, *C* and *D*).

Current Problem and Management

At 3-month follow-up, slight loss of correction with screw breakage was evident at both the femoral and the tibial tubercle osteotomy sites, and delayed union was seen on the tibial side (**Figure 8**). At 6-month follow-up, the femoral osteotomy showed complete healing, but both the high tibial and tibial tubercle osteotomies had progressed to nonunion.

The patient underwent revision surgery on her right knee. The patellar tendon and the tibial tubercle, which had pulled off the tibia, were identified. Fibrous scar tissue between the tibial tubercle fragment and the anterior tibia was débrided. All hardware, including the plate and screws from the tibial osteotomy and the three screws from the tibial tubercle osteotomy, were removed. The osteotomy was débrided of all soft-tissue debris and the tissue was sent for culture. A thorough irrigation was performed with pulsatile lavage. The osteotomy site was packed with cancellous bone chips both anterior and posterior to the 90° blade plate that was used for revision fixation.

To reapproximate the tibial tubercle, three anchors were placed in the anterior tibia, and the sutures were pulled up through the remnants of the tibial tubercle and patellar tendon in a horizontal mattress configuration (**Figure 9**). Examination of the knee after fixation revealed a range of motion of approximately 0° to 100°.

Outcome

At latest follow-up, the patient had no pain, had good range of motion, and was able to ambulate for activities of daily living.

Discussion

Recognizing the Problem

In this case, two main complications occurred: fracture of the medial hinge on the femur and nonunion of the proximal tibia.

© 2011 American Academy of Orthopaedic Surgeons

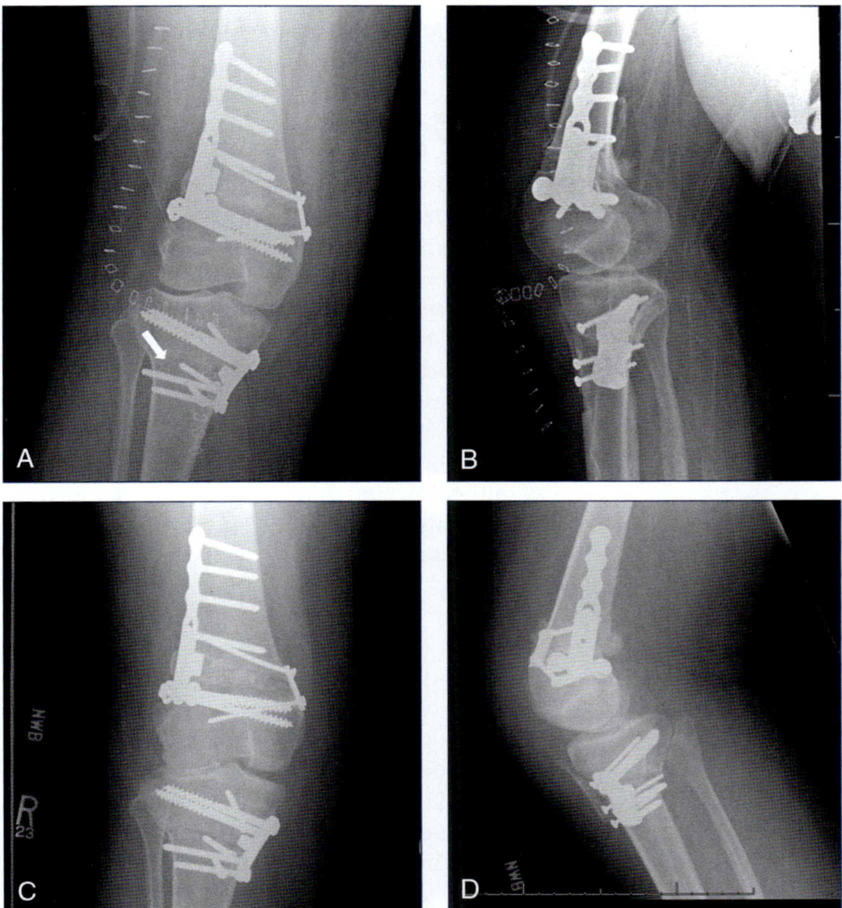

Figure 7 Postoperative images of the right knee of the same patient shown in Figure 5. She underwent surgery that included opening wedge HTO in conjunction with opening wedge DFO, patellectomy, and extensor mechanism distal realignment in the right knee 1 year after surgery on the left knee. AP (**A**) and lateral (**B**) radiographs show a medial femoral hinge disruption stabilized intraoperatively with a two-hole plate. Note the fracture line directed distally from the tibial osteotomy site (arrow), which was not recognized on intraoperative fluoroscopy. AP (**C**) and lateral (**D**) radiographs obtained at 6-week follow-up show proximal migration of the tibial tubercle with no loss of correction and no hardware breakage

Fracture is one of the most common intraoperative complications in HTO/DFO. The rate of lateral cortex fracture during medial opening wedge HTO has been reported to be as high as 12%.[13] The fracture can be either intra-articular or extra-articular medial/lateral hinge disruption.

Managing the Problem

If an intra-articular or extra-articular fracture occurs, it should be recognized intraoperatively and addressed. The stability of the osteotomy can be checked manually with varus/valgus stress maneuvers, but fluoroscopy remains the most valuable tool in the early recognition of fracture.

Intra-articular fractures usually are not displaced, but they require fixation in addition to the osteotomy plate. Of the many techniques available, percutaneous screw fixation generally ensures good stability.[14] Lag screws can be introduced parallel to the joint line either medially or laterally, according to the fracture pattern. Intra-articular fractures require a less aggressive rehabilitation protocol, with 2 months of non–weight bearing and range of motion restricted to 0° to 90° range of motion for at least 1 month.

Extra-articular fractures most commonly include disruption of the medial or lateral hinge. A stable osteotomy fixation is essential to reduce the risk of loss of correction and nonunion. The many techniques used to restore medial/lateral hinge stability include lag screw fixation, two-hole plate or staple fixation,[13] and long locking-plate osteotomy fixation.[14] In opening wedge osteotomies, locking plates have the advantage that no further procedures are required to restore the disrupted hinge.[15] On the

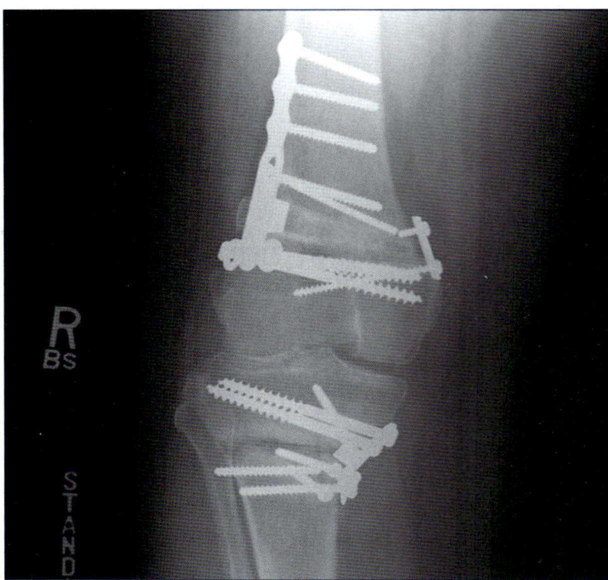

Figure 8 Weight-bearing AP radiograph of the same knee shown in Figure 7 obtained at 3-month follow-up shows healing and one broken screw on the femoral side and developing nonunion and hardware failure on the tibial side.

other hand, locking plates have a high profile, are less tolerated by patients, and often require hardware removal. A conventional plate, however, has the disadvantage that the disrupted hinge has to be stabilized.[14] Fixation can be achieved by using both a two-hole plate and staples and lag screws placed opposite the osteotomy plate.[14]

If the hinge disruption is recognized postoperatively, a cautious rehabilitation protocol (one that prolongs the non–weight-bearing phase until radiographic evidence of osteotomy healing is seen) should be considered. In most cases, this management avoids loss of correction and nonunion. If only slight loss of correction occurs (3° to 5°), the patient's symptoms should guide the decision to consider revision.

The incidence of nonunion is 1.6% in medial opening wedge osteotomy[5] and 0.5% to 5.7% in lateral closing wedge osteotomy.[3] Proper patient selection (see Case 1 Discussion), stable fixation, and appropriate gap filling (with correction >10°) are essential to prevent nonunion. Revision is always indicated in nonunion and usually includes hardware removal, fibrous tissue débridement, and new fixation with a different device, performed with or without autologous bone grafting.

Preventing the Problem

The surgical technique for HTO/DFO must be accurate and precise to prevent intra-articular or extra-articular fractures. Use of a guidewire to assess the osteotomy line and to drive the chisels is mandatory. The osteotomes should be placed below (HTO) or above (DFO) the Kirschner wire to avoid directing the osteotomy line into the joint. The length of the bone cut should be planned based on the preoperative radiographs and carefully checked on the graduated osteotomes during surgery to preserve the medial/lateral hinge. Also, the anterior and posterior cortices must be completely cut, and the medial/lateral hinge must be preserved. Before inserting the wedges and opening the osteotomy, it is important to apply a valgus (HTO) or varus (DFO) stress on the knee joint and to visualize a slight (about 5-mm) opening of the osteotomy site. If the osteotomy site does not open, the bone cut is probably incomplete at the anterior or posterior cortex and must be addressed. Another method that can minimize the risk of fractures is the "three-osteotome technique," in which two osteotomes are inserted into the osteotomy, one above the other, and a third osteotome is inserted between them. This technique can allow a gradual and progressive opening at the osteotomy site.

Strategies to Minimize Common Complications

In a recent study by the University of Iowa Hospitals and Clinics,[16] the incidence of major and minor complications was analyzed in a total of 62 knee osteotomies performed from 2001 to 2005. The cohort consisted of 46 HTOs and 16 DFOs. The average follow-up time was 15.7 months (range, 1.3 to 50.2 months) for HTO patients and 14.3 months (range, 3.1 to 40.2 months) for DFO patients. Knee osteotomy was performed with additional reconstructive procedures (cruciate or collateral ligament reconstruction, meniscal transplantation, cartilage resurfacing using osteochondral allograft or autograft transplantation or autologous chondrocyte

© 2011 American Academy of Orthopaedic Surgeons

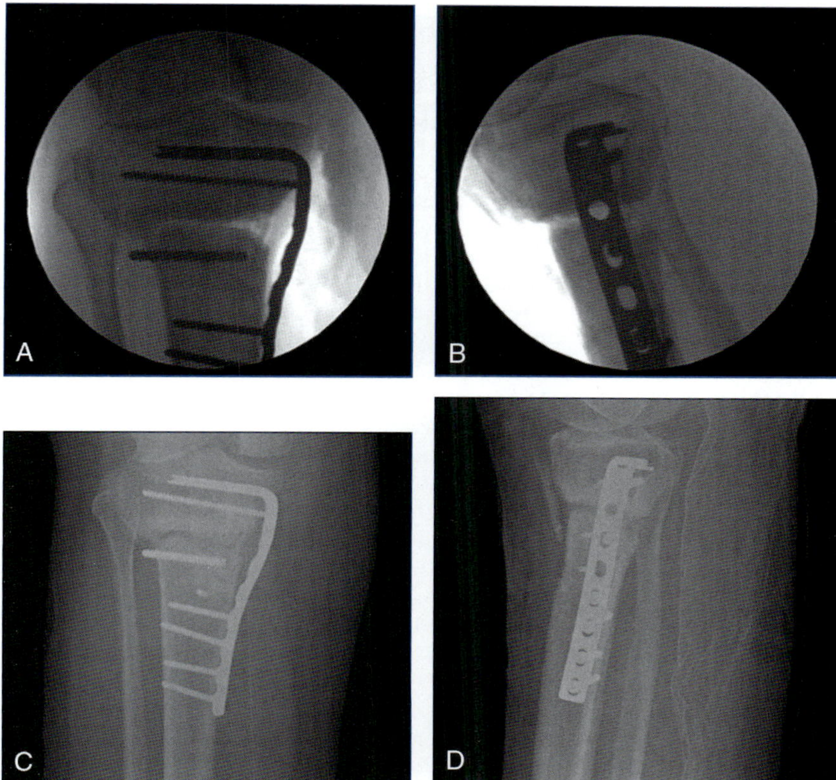

Figure 9 Images of the same knee shown in Figures 7 and 8. Intraoperative AP (**A**) and lateral (**B**) fluoroscopic views obtained after hardware removal (except for the broken screw) and revision fixation with a 90° blade plate. Postoperative AP (**C**) and lateral (**D**) radiographs show the new fixation and reduction of the tibial tubercle.

implantation, or patellar realignment) in 39.1% of HTO patients and 62.5% of DFO patients. Patients who underwent a combined procedure were significantly younger than patients who underwent only osteotomy (27.9 versus 40.1 years; $P < 0.001$). Major complications were found in 19.6% of HTO patients and 25.0% of DFO patients. Minor complications were found in 39.1% of HTO patients and 18.8% of DFO patients. Major complications were found in 25.0% of patients who underwent an additional procedure with a knee osteotomy and 17.6% of patients who underwent only osteotomy, but this difference was not statistically significant. These data show that in HTO and DFO, the rates for minor complications are also high and every effort should be made to minimize the risks.

Infection

The combined deep and superficial infection rates range from 2.3% to 54.4%.[14] The higher risk is associated with external fixators, but the infection is usually superficial, is limited to the pin tract, and mostly responds to oral antibiotics. In osteotomies stabilized with internal fixation, the risk is generally less than 4%.[17] Intravenous antibiotic prophylaxis for minor orthopaedic surgery should be administered (ie, first-generation cephalosporin [2 g of cefazoline in 100 mL saline administered 10 minutes before incision]). Careful skin preparation and disinfection also should be performed.

Patella Infera or Patella Alta

Before the use of internal fixation and early motion in HTO, when cast immobilization was part of the postoperative treatment, authors reported a 7.6% to 8.8% risk of patella infera following a lateral closing wedge HTO.[4] This complication probably was due to contracture of the patellar tendon during immobilization. A more recent study[18] showed that closing wedge HTO and opening wedge DFO combined

© 2011 American Academy of Orthopaedic Surgeons

increase patellar height by lowering the joint line. On the other hand, opening wedge HTO and closing wedge DFO decrease patellar height by raising the joint line. Accurate preoperative evaluation of patellar height can avoid the risk of patella infera and patella alta. The implications of patellar height changes for clinical outcomes are still controversial.

Compartment Syndrome

Although compartment syndrome has been described as a complication of HTO, its exact incidence is not known.[19] Some authors suggest using a drain to reduce compartment pressures,[20] and others have reported an increased risk with associated arthroscopic ligament reconstruction.[21]

Peroneal Nerve Palsy

Peroneal nerve palsy due to direct injury is a complication described for closing wedge HTO; its incidence ranges from 2% to 16%.[4] If the fibular osteotomy is performed more than 15 cm distal to the head, this risk is reduced. Nonetheless, neurologic complications after medial opening wedge HTO have been reported.[4]

Thromboembolism

The incidence of deep vein thrombosis (DVT) ranges from 1.3% to 9.8%,[4] and fatal pulmonary embolism has been reported.[22] Prophylaxis with low-molecular-weight heparin is a valuable measure to reduce the rate of DVT. Diagnosis of DVT using Doppler ultrasonography of the calf and adequate therapy performed early are important.

Other Complications

Other complications include pseudarthrosis of the fibula (only in closing wedge HTO), vascular injuries, necrosis of the proximal tibia, and failure of fixation with or without loss of correction.[4] For most of these complications, the exact incidences are not available and they are described mainly in case reports.[4]

References

1. Akizuki S, Shibakawa A, Takizawa T, Yamazaki I, Horiuchi H: The long-term outcome of high tibial osteotomy: A ten- to 20-year follow-up. *J Bone Joint Surg Br* 2008;90(5):592-596.
2. Flecher X, Parratte S, Aubaniac JM, Argenson JN: A 12-28-year followup study of closing wedge high tibial osteotomy. *Clin Orthop Relat Res* 2006(452):91-96.
3. Amendola A, Bonasia DE: Results of high tibial osteotomy: Review of the literature. *Int Orthop* 2010;34(2):155-160.
4. Amendola A, Bonasia DE: Results of HTO in medial OA of the knee, in Amendola A, Bellemans J, Bonnin M, MacDonald S, Menetrey J, eds: *The Knee Joint: Surgical Techniques and Strategies.* (in press)
5. Warden SJ, Morris HG, Crossley KM, Brukner PD, Bennell KL: Delayed- and non-union following opening wedge high tibial osteotomy: Surgeons' results from 182 completed cases. *Knee Surg Sports Traumatol Arthrosc* 2005;13(1):34-37.
6. Amendola A: Unicompartmental osteoarthritis in the active patient: The role of high tibial osteotomy. *Arthroscopy* 2003;19(10 Suppl 1)109-116.
7. Aryee S, Imhoff AB, Rose T, Tischer T: Do we need synthetic osteotomy augmentation materials for opening-wedge high tibial osteotomy. *Biomaterials* 2008;29(26): 3497-3502.
8. Dallari D, Savarino L, Stagni C, et al: Enhanced tibial osteotomy healing with use of bone grafts supplemented with platelet gel or platelet gel and bone marrow stromal cells. *J Bone Joint Surg Am* 2007;89(11): 2413-2420.
9. Eid K, Zelicof S, Perona BP, Sledge CB, Glowacki J: Tissue reactions to particles of bone-substitute materials in intraosseous and heterotopic sites in rats: Discrimination of osteoinduction, osteocompatibility, and inflammation. *J Orthop Res* 2001;19(5):962-969.
10. Gaasbeek RD, Toonen HG, van Heerwaarden RJ, Buma P: Mechanism of bone incorporation of beta-TCP bone substitute in open wedge tibial osteotomy in patients. *Biomaterials* 2005;26(33):6713-6719.
11. LeGeros RZ: Properties of osteoconductive biomaterials: Calcium phosphates. *Clin Orthop Relat Res* 2002(395):81-98.
12. Hernigou P, Ma W: Open wedge tibial osteotomy with acrylic bone cement as bone substitute. *Knee* 2001; 8(2):103-110.

© 2011 American Academy of Orthopaedic Surgeons

13. Kazimoğlu C, Akdoğan Y, Şener M, Kurtulmuş A, Karapınar H, Uzun B: Which is the best fixation method for lateral cortex disruption in the medial open wedge high tibial osteotomy? A biomechanical study. *Knee* 2008;15(4):305-308.
14. Spahn G: Complications in high tibial (medial opening wedge) osteotomy. *Arch Orthop Trauma Surg* 2004; 124(10):649-653.
15. Agneskirchner JD, Freiling D, Hurschler C, Lobenhoffer P: Primary stability of four different implants for opening wedge high tibial osteotomy. *Knee Surg Sports Traumatol Arthrosc* 2006;14(3):291-300.
16. Willey M, Wolf BR, Kocaglu B, Amendola A: Complications associated with realignment osteotomy of the knee performed simultaneously with additional reconstructive procedures. *Iowa Orthop J* 2010;30: 55-60.
17. Billings A, Scott DF, Camargo MP, Hofmann AA: High tibial osteotomy with a calibrated osteotomy guide, rigid internal fixation, and early motion: Long-term follow-up. *J Bone Joint Surg Am* 2000;82(1):70-79.
18. Wright JM, Heavrin B, Begg M, Sakyrd G, Sterett W: Observations on patellar height following opening wedge proximal tibial osteotomy. *Am J Knee Surg* 2001;14(3):163-173.
19. Wright JM, Crockett HC, Slawski DP, Madsen MW, Windsor RE: High tibial osteotomy. *J Am Acad Orthop Surg* 2005;13(4):279-289.
20. Gibson MJ, Barnes MR, Allen MJ, Chan RN: Weakness of foot dorsiflexion and changes in compartment pressures after tibial osteotomy. *J Bone Joint Surg Br* 1986;68(3):471-475.
21. Marti CB, Jakob RP: Accumulation of irrigation fluid in the calf as a complication during high tibial osteotomy combined with simultaneous arthroscopic anterior cruciate ligament reconstruction. *Arthroscopy* 1999;15(8): 864-866.
22. Insall JN, Joseph DM, Msika C: High tibial osteotomy for varus gonarthrosis: A long-term follow-up study. *J Bone Joint Surg Am* 1984;66(7):1040-1048.

Chapter 6

Meniscal Allograft Transplantation

Nicole A. Friel, MS
Shane J. Nho, MD, MS
Joseph U. Barker, MD
Vasili Karas, MS
Brian J. Cole, MD, MBA

Introduction

The meniscus is a critical structure in the knee, and its role in shock absorption,[1] load transmission,[2] secondary mechanical stability,[3] joint lubrication,[4] and nutrition[5] is well documented. As such, orthopaedic surgeons prefer to repair and preserve the meniscus whenever possible. When patients who have undergone high-grade knee meniscectomy become symptomatic, meniscal allograft transplantation can be considered to decrease pain and improve function. Several techniques for meniscal allograft transplantation have been described.[6-8] This chapter discusses the appropriate diagnosis and treatment of the most common complications, as well as strategies to minimize their occurrence.

Case 1: Articular Cartilage Defect

History

A 25-year-old woman had undergone multiple knee surgeries including two anterior cruciate ligament (ACL) reconstructions, three partial medial meniscectomies, and a medial meniscal transplantation. The patient's early postoperative course following meniscal transplantation was unremarkable.

Current Problem

At 12-month follow-up, the patient reported medial-side pain and a minimal effusion. MRI obtained 12 months postoperatively demonstrated a new focal chondral defect with bone edema in the medial femoral condyle.

Dr. Nho or an immediate family member has received research or institutional support from Arthrex, DJ Orthopaedics, Linvatec, Össur, Smith & Nephew, Athletico, and Miomed. Dr. Cole or an immediate family member has received royalties from Arthrex; serves as a paid consultant to or is an employee of Genzyme, Zimmer, DePuy, Arthrex, Carticept, and Regentis; and has received research or institutional support from Arthrex, DePuy, Zimmer, Genzyme, and DJ Orthopaedics. None of the following authors nor any immediate family member has received anything of value from or owns stock in a commercial company or institution related directly or indirectly to the subject of this chapter: Ms. Friel, Dr. Barker, and Mr. Karas.

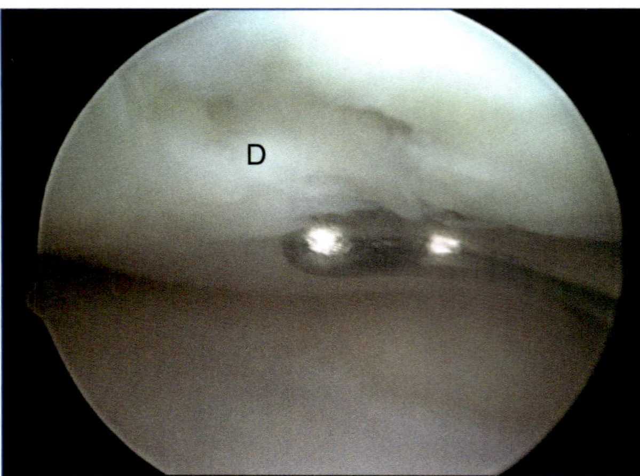

Figure 1 Arthroscopic image of the knee of the 25-year-old woman described in case 1, who had undergone multiple knee surgeries, shows a focal chondral defect (D) of the medial femoral condyle measuring 12 × 12 mm following medial meniscal transplantation.

Management

Arthroscopy demonstrated an intact medial meniscus and a focal cartilage defect of the medial femoral condyle measuring 12 × 12 mm (**Figure 1**). The cartilage lesion was treated with microfracture.

Outcome

The patient did well immediately following surgery. At 1-year follow-up, the patient experienced intermittent pain that she described as aching, but she was mostly satisfied with the outcome at the time. Although she was unable to participate in sports that called for jumping and twisting, she was able to participate in light running. Upon physical examination, the patient exhibited full range of motion and a stable knee.

Case 2: Articular Cartilage Defect

History

A 40-year-old man with a history of gout had undergone four arthroscopic lateral meniscectomies and presented with worsening lateral knee pain and mild effusion. Prior to the onset of symptoms, this patient was active, playing tennis one to two times per week. Diagnostic arthroscopy demonstrated an absent lateral meniscus with a 20 × 20–mm chondral defect of the lateral femoral condyle. The patient was diagnosed with lateral compartment meniscal deficiency with a focal chondral defect of the lateral femoral condyle.

Management

The patient underwent concurrent lateral meniscal allograft transplantation and osteochondral allograft transplantation of the lateral femoral condyle with a 20 × 20–mm plug (**Figure 2**).

Outcome

The patient did well following surgery and at 3-year follow-up, but he reported occasional pain when jogging or walking for extended periods of time. He resumed sporting activities one to two times per week. The patient did report occasional effusion after activity, which resolved when treated with ice, rest, and anti-inflammatory medication.

Discussion

Degenerative changes and full-thickness chondral defects historically have been considered a contraindication for meniscal transplantation because of disappointing clinical outcomes. Recently, several studies have shown excellent results in carefully selected patients when meniscal allograft transplantation was performed concurrently with autologous chondrocyte implantation[9-11] or osteochondral allograft transplantation.[11] Cases 1 and 2 demonstrate the importance of assessing and treating chondral damage associated with meniscal deficiency to maximize outcomes.

Case 1 is an example of a patient with early localized cartilage degeneration occurring after meniscal transplantation. Left untreated, as the chondral defect progresses, the joint becomes more hostile for the meniscal allograft, which can lead to excessive stress on the transplanted meniscus, causing subsequent degeneration. The focal chondral defect in case 1 was found during diagnostic arthroscopy following meniscal transplantation. The small size of the lesion aided in the decision to treat with microfracture during the arthroscopy rather than plan a second, larger procedure such as osteochon-

© 2011 *American Academy of Orthopaedic Surgeons*

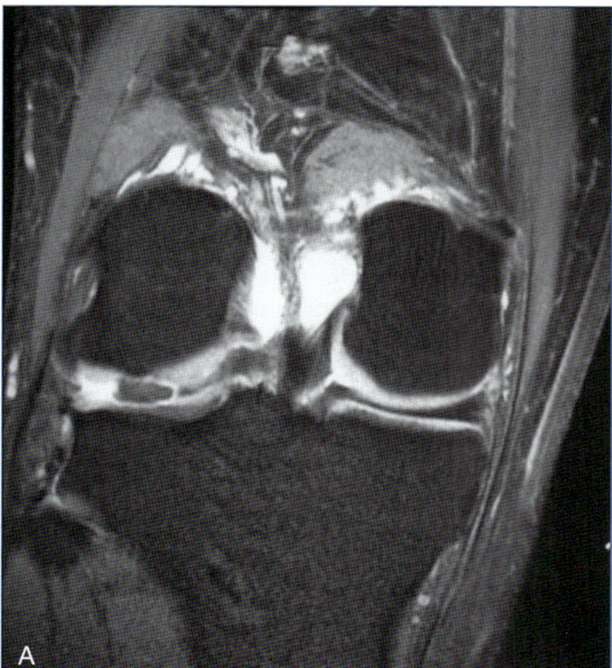

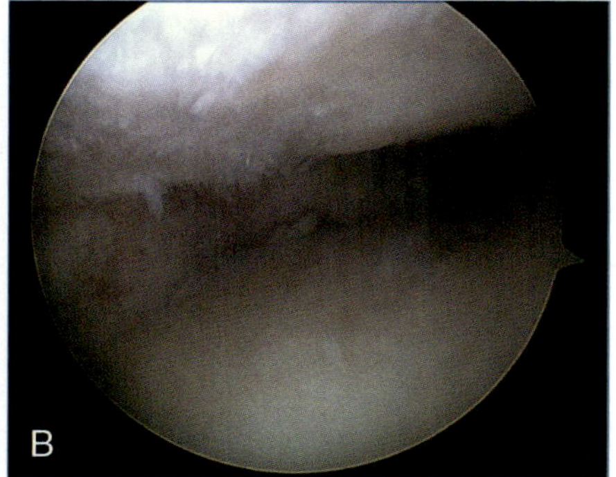

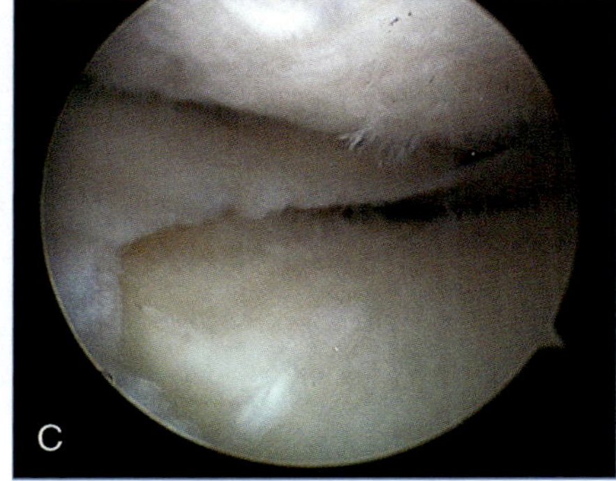

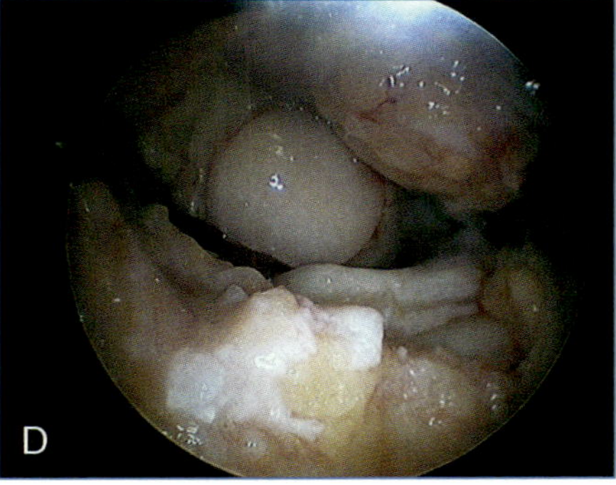

Figure 2 Images of the knee of the 40-year-old man described in case 2, who had undergone four knee surgeries. **A,** T2-weighted coronal MRI demonstrates deficient lateral meniscus with cartilage defect of the lateral femoral condyle. **B,** Arthroscopic image of the lateral compartment demonstrates meniscal deficiency with a grade III International Cartilage Repair Society chondral defect of the lateral femoral condyle. **C,** Arthroscopic image of the transplanted lateral meniscus shows a persistent cartilage lesion. **D,** Intraoperative arthroscopic image shows a fresh osteochondral allograft measuring 20 × 20 mm implanted in the lateral femoral condyle.

dral allograft transplantation or autologous chondrocyte implantation. When chondral defects are detected before the meniscal transplantation, as in case 2, they should be repaired in concurrent or staged procedures to address all joint pathology. In case 2, previous arthroscopy had revealed a large focal defect. Given the size and location of the defect, it was treated with an osteochondral allograft concurrently with the meniscal transplantation.

Similarly, if malalignment is demonstrated on long-leg weight-bearing radiographs, concomitant osteotomy, cartilage restoration, and meniscal transplantation can be planned preoperatively.[12] Axial malalignment can exert increased contact pressure on any cartilage-deficient areas as well as on the newly placed graft, which can lead to overload, loosening, degeneration, and failure. Concurrent or staged corrective osteotomy is indicated in patients in whom the mechanical axis falls in the involved compartment. The goal of correction depends on the degree of chondral damage. Often, correction of malalignment to a weight-bearing line that falls between the tibial spines is adequate. If larger chondral defects are present, however, a mild degree of overcorrection can be preferable, with a weight-bearing line that falls just outside the contralateral tibial spine.[13]

When meniscal transplantation is performed concomitant with a cartilage restoration procedure, it is generally safer and easier to perform all steps of the meniscal transplantation first and then proceed with the cartilage restoration procedure. Special care should be taken to avoid damaging the anterior horn of the transplanted meniscus when creating the arthrotomy required for the cartilage restoration procedure (ie, autologous chondrocyte implantation or osteochondral allograft transplantation). Keeping the knee in a flexed position, meticulous dissection, and careful soft-tissue retraction can prevent damage.

Case 3: Ligamentous Instability and Meniscal Deficiency

History

A 16-year-old boy underwent a left-knee ACL reconstruction with a quadriceps tendon autograft and subtotal medial and lateral meniscectomy.

Current Problem

At 2-year postoperative presentation, the patient reported that the knee was normal with routine activities of daily living but he experienced swelling and pain localized to the medial aspect of the knee after strenuous activities. The patient had not been able to participate in basketball or any sports activities since the most recent surgery. The patient also reported episodes of giving way and knee apprehension. The patient denied having mechanical symptoms, anterior knee pain, or any difficulties with stair climbing. The patient was diagnosed with ligament instability in a meniscus-deficient knee.

Management

The patient was treated with concomitant medial meniscal transplantation and revision ACL reconstruction.

Outcome

The patient had no postoperative complications and successfully completed his rehabilitation protocol. He returned to his previous level of activity (prior to index ACL reconstruction) after 9 months. Physical examination showed a stable knee without tenderness along the joint line bilaterally. Although it does not illustrate a direct complication of meniscal allograft transplantation, this case serves an educational purpose and demonstrates the high-level decision making related to meniscal allograft transplantation and coexisting ACL pathology.

Discussion

A relatively common indication for medial meniscal allograft transplantation is recurrent instability following previous ACL reconstruction in the meniscectomized knee. Because the menisci serve as secondary stabilizers to anterior-posterior translation of the knee, an ACL-reconstructed knee relies on the medial meniscus to play a protective role. In addition, combined ACL and meniscal deficiency has a poor prognosis because of the frequent development of secondary arthritis over time. The surgical technique for combined ACL reconstruction and medial meniscal allograft transplantation is difficult because of the risk of complications associated with overlap between the tibial tunnel and meniscal slot placement. The preferred method for the meniscal allograft preparation is a modified bridge-in-slot technique: the bone block is cut into thirds, the anterior and posterior blocks (with their respective meniscal insertions) are preserved and prepared with nonabsorbable transosseous sutures, and the middle bone block is discarded. A vertical mattress traction suture (No. 0 polydioxanone [PDS]) is placed at the junction of the posterior horn and the middle third of the meniscus (**Figure 3**, *A*). Our preferred ACL graft for the combined procedure is an Achilles tendon allograft because it has no bone block in the tibia that potentially can interfere with the slot for the meniscal allograft.

The tibial tunnel for the ACL is drilled first, followed by the creation of the femoral tunnel. The tibial tunnel should be drilled as obliquely as possible, entering the lateral aspect of the tibial footprint to minimize interference with the bone trough for the meniscus.

© 2011 American Academy of Orthopaedic Surgeons

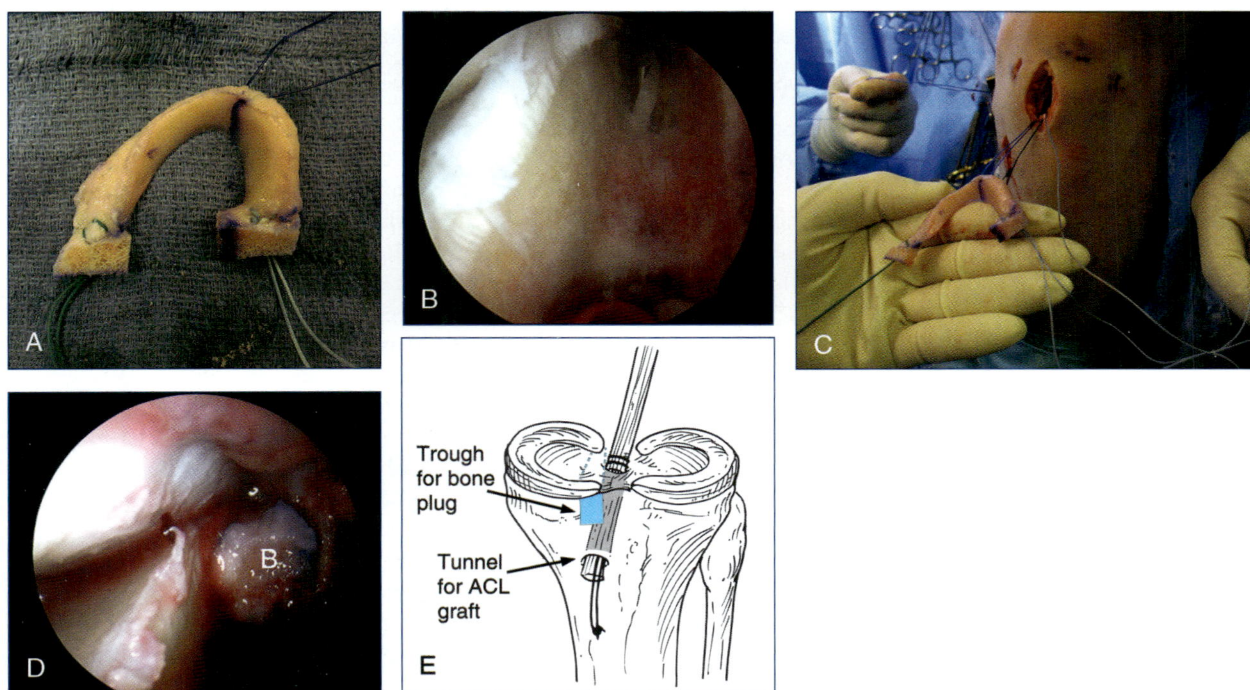

Figure 3 Images illustrate medial meniscal transplantation in a 16-year-old boy (case 3). **A,** Photograph of a prepared meniscal allograft shows one traction suture placed at the junction between the posterior and middle thirds of the meniscus. The anterior and posterior bone blocks are secured with a transosseous braided, nonabsorbable suture. **B,** Arthroscopic view of the meniscal trough. The tibial tunnel for the ACL can be seen at the bottom (red), and the tibial tunnel for the posterior horn fixation can be seen at the top. **C,** Intraoperative photograph shows preparation for seating the meniscal transplant. **D,** Arthroscopic view of the bone trough shows proper placement of the posterior bone block (B) within the bone trough. **E,** Drawing of the completed medial meniscal transplantation and ACL reconstruction shows the relationship between the ACL tibial tunnel, the meniscal bone trough, and suture fixation for the anterior and posterior bone blocks.

The bone trough should be completed as it would be for isolated medial meniscal transplantation, using the bridge-in-slot technique. The bone trough is made through the lateral aspect of the medial tibial plateau to accept the allograft bone bridge. Following creation of the trough, a transtibial ACL guide is used to create two small transosseous tunnels, one in each of the anterior and posterior aspects of the trough, for subsequent fixation of the respective anterior and posterior bone blocks of the meniscal allograft. Two suture shuttles are placed within these transosseous tunnels to facilitate graft suture passage (**Figure 3,** *B*).

The posterior aspect of the meniscal allograft is placed into the slot before the ACL graft is placed (**Figure 3,** *C*). The sutures on the posterior bone block are passed through the posterior transosseous tibial tunnel. With the aid of the traction sutures, the meniscal allograft is gently pulled (and pushed) into the joint through the anterior arthrotomy while the posterior bone block is advanced into the tibial slot and pulled into place (**Figure 3,** *D*). The meniscus is manually reduced under the condyle with a finger placed through the arthrotomy and a valgus force placed on the knee joint. Leading with the bone block, the ACL graft is passed through the tibia and

© 2011 *American Academy of Orthopaedic Surgeons*

into the femur just anterior to the posterior bone block that is seated in the tibial trough (bone plug–free central area). The anterior bone block then is secured into place by pulling the sutures through the anterior tibial bone tunnel. The posterior and anterior transosseous fixation sutures are tied over a bone bridge or suture button, securing the bone blocks. The meniscus then is repaired using multiple inside-out vertical mattress sutures. An illustration of the completed meniscus transplant and ACL reconstruction is provided in **Figure 3**, *E*.

Case 4: Intraoperative Compromised Bone Block Fixation

History

A 20-year-old man who had undergone an arthroscopic partial lateral meniscectomy presented with persistent lateral joint line pain and was recommended for lateral meniscal transplant. During the procedure, the bone trough was appropriately prepared and the bone block was inserted. The graft was positioned in the slot, and a 7 × 25–mm biocomposite interference screw was used to secure the bone plug in place. The peripheral sutures were placed to secure the meniscus to the capsule. After the peripheral sutures were completed, it was noted that the screw and bone block had dislodged out of the tibial trough.

Management

The initial screw was replaced with a larger biocomposite interference screw (8 × 28 mm). This was performed while the block was held firmly reduced in the trough using an elevator introduced through the arthrotomy. Full extension of the leg did not cause impingement, and the graft was stable throughout range of motion.

Outcome

The patient recovered from surgery and had no further complications. Radiographs were obtained immediately postoperatively and showed proper placement of the interference screw and bone block. At 2-year follow-up, the patient had resumed previous levels of activity, which included light athletic activity two to three times per week.

Discussion

Secure fixation of the bone block is critical to the successful placement of the meniscal allograft. The bone bridge normally is secured within the tibial slot with a biocomposite interference screw. Inadequate screw fixation that does not allow proper seating of the graft can be remedied in several ways. In this case, the screw was removed and replaced with a larger screw to improve fixation.

Although the bone block provides additional stability, better load transmission biomechanics, and improved bone-to-bone healing, placement of the bone block into the trough can be a tight fit, and fracture of the bone block can occur. If the bone block fractures, the surgeon can convert to transosseous suture fixation as described previously. Additionally, if the bone block breaks after the interference screw is placed and the posterior aspect of the bone block is secure, the anterior bone block can be secured with either a separate interference screw or transosseous suture fixation through a tibial tunnel. If the bone is compromised at either the anterior or posterior horn, soft-tissue fixation placed transosseously through the tibia also can be used.

Case 5: Torn Meniscal Allograft

History

A 44-year-old man underwent lateral meniscal allograft transplantation for persistent knee pain following a lateral meniscectomy 2 years prior. Prior to the onset of knee symptoms, the patient was active, playing basketball or running four to five times per week. One year after meniscal transplantation, he returned to biking and running.

Current Problem

The patient sustained a twisting event to the knee 27 months after the index procedure. He presented to the clinic with recurrent pain. MRI showed evidence of a tear of the lateral meniscal allograft (**Figure 4**, *A*). Arthroscopy confirmed a displaced bucket-

© 2011 American Academy of Orthopaedic Surgeons

handle tear in the peripheral third of the meniscus extending posteriorly to the popliteal hiatus (**Figure 4**, *B*). The meniscus was completely torn and avulsed from the capsule. Otherwise, the meniscus showed no degeneration. The patient was diagnosed with a meniscal allograft tear.

Management

Débridement, meniscectomy, meniscal repair, and revision meniscal transplantation all were considered in the treatment of this patient. The option chosen depends on the characteristics of the tear and the response of the patient to initial treatment. Because this patient did well following the index meniscal transplantation until the traumatic event occurred, he was treated with meniscal repair.

Outcome

The patient was symptom-free at follow-up. He returned to the level of activity achieved after the index procedure.

Discussion

Tears of meniscal allografts are treated similarly to tears of the native meniscus. Meniscal transplant repair should be attempted for tears in the peripheral third (red-red zone). The repaired meniscus may not heal, however; the rate and success of healing of a repaired meniscal allograft has not been established. The surgeon should attempt to optimize the local biologic environment by rasping the torn surfaces and synovium and should consider using a fibrin clot, marrow stimulation, and/or platelet-rich plasma.[14] Tears located in the middle and inner thirds should be carefully excised and contoured to the surrounding meniscus. If the patient remains symptomatic after partial meniscectomy, revision meniscal allograft transplantation should be considered, especially if the patient tolerated the initial transplant but then sustained a traumatic tear.

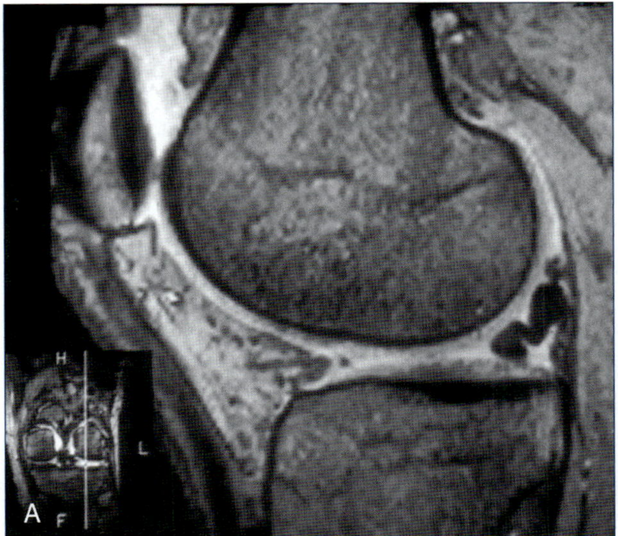

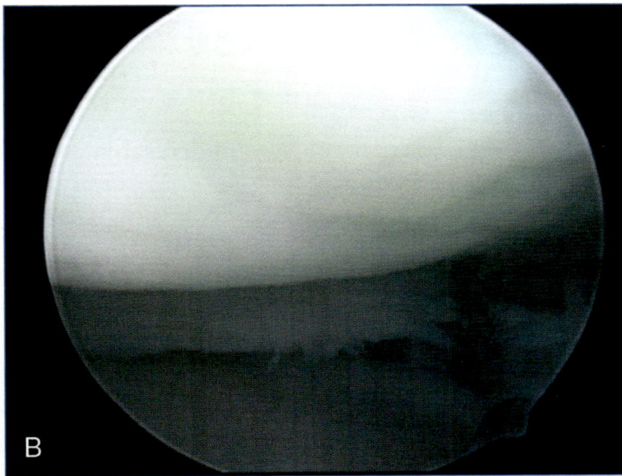

Figure 4 Images obtained at 27-month follow-up of the knee of the 44-year-old man described in case 5. The patient underwent lateral meniscal allograft transplantation after a twisting event. **A,** Sagittal T2-weighted MRI suggests a tear of the meniscus. Lower-left inset shows line indicating location of image section on coronal view. **B,** Arthroscopic view shows a displaced bucket-handle tear in the meniscal allograft extending posteriorly to the popliteal hiatus.

© 2011 *American Academy of Orthopaedic Surgeons*

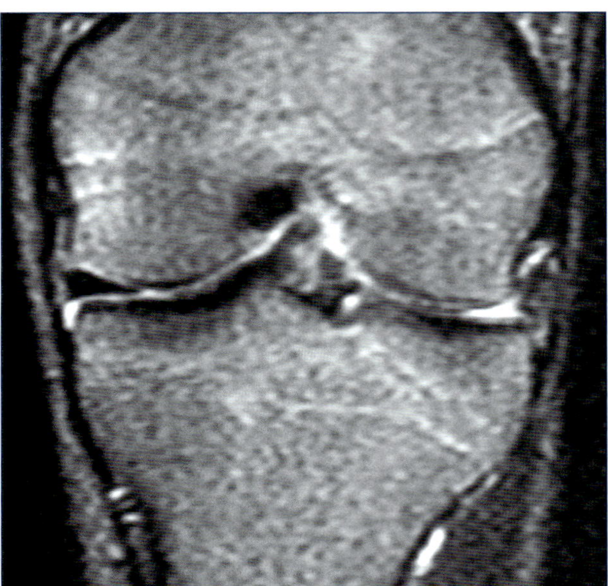

Figure 5 Coronal T2-weighted MRI of the knee of the 25-year-old woman described in case 6, obtained 6 months after lateral meniscal allograft transplantation. Note the extrusion of the lateral menisus.

Case 6: Postoperative Meniscal Subluxation

History

A 25-year-old woman underwent lateral meniscal allograft transplantation. Her symptoms improved, but she was never completely without pain.

Current Problem

Lateral joint line tenderness developed, and an MRI obtained at 6-month follow-up demonstrated lateral extrusion of the meniscus (**Figure 5**). The patient also reported a feeling of instability. The patient was diagnosed with lateral subluxation of the meniscus.

Management

The patient underwent a revision meniscal transplantation, which is the ideal treatment for symptomatic extrusion of a meniscal transplant. In light of her symptoms as well as the MRI findings, she elected to undergo revision mensical transplantation.

Outcome

At 6-month follow-up, the patient was able to return to full activity. At 1-year follow-up, the patient still reported mild pain as well as occasional swelling. Her instability, however, improved. Physical examination showed no effusion, active range of motion from 0° to 130°, and mild tenderness over the posterolateral joint line.

Discussion

Meniscal subluxation can be identified on MRI. Extrusion of the meniscus is concerning, because it compromises the meniscus in load transmission and shock absorption and can lead to secondary mechanical instability. Studies of meniscal subluxation in nontransplanted patients have shown an association between meniscal subluxation and joint space narrowing and symptomatic osteoarthritis.[15,16] Some outcome studies on meniscal transplantation, however, have shown no correlation between allograft extrusion and clinical outcome.[17,18] Therefore, only symptomatic patients should be considered for revision transplantation. Further studies are needed to determine long-term outcomes of untreated extruded meniscal transplants.

Although the cause of meniscal extrusion is not known, extrusion is thought to result from graft size mismatch or from excessively tight meniscocapsular sutures. Securing the rim of the allograft to the capsular tissue using inside-out vertical mattress sutures is important for fixation, but pulling the graft too far toward the capsule can compromise correct anatomic positioning. In addition, excessive débridement and inadvertent capsulectomy during preparation for the transplant can lead to extrusion.

Case 7: Meniscal Shrinkage

History

A 31-year-old woman underwent medial meniscal allograft transplantation and ACL thermal shrinkage after a traumatic tear of the meniscus during athletic activity.

Current Problem

The patient presented to the clinic 8 years postoperatively with medial-side knee pain and subtle insta-

© 2011 American Academy of Orthopaedic Surgeons

bility. Physical examination showed significant tenderness along the posteromedial joint line and a grade 1 pivot-shift test (a twisting slide with the tibia twisting internally). MRI demonstrated grossly intact articular surfaces but a shrunken meniscus. Diagnostic arthroscopy revealed meniscal shrinkage and minor fissuring on the meniscal undersurface but no frank tears of the allograft. The patient was diagnosed with failed primary meniscal transplantation secondary to meniscal shrinkage and ultrastructural failure.

Management

The patient was treated with revision meniscal transplantation because she had a very good outcome for 7 years following the initial meniscal transplantation and did not fare well with meniscectomy.

Outcome

The patient was pain-free 1 year postoperatively. She returned to her previous level of activity with the exception of running, which caused minimal swelling of the knee.

Discussion

Revision meniscal transplantation is a viable option in a young patient with realistic goals who has recovered well from the index procedure but has experienced a traumatic event or acute increase of pain and decrease in function.

The surgical technique for the revision procedure varies, but any index surgery generally can be revised using a bridge-in-slot technique. This technique allows adequate rigid bony fixation and maintains the native anterior and posterior meniscal horn attachments. Using a bridge-in-slot technique for the revision, however, may require enlargement of the original slot back to fresh bleeding bone, thereby using a slightly larger meniscal bone bridge, which may increase the relative morbidity of the surgical procedure.[19]

The procedure for revision using a bridge-in-slot technique is nearly identical to the index procedure. The previous meniscal bone block is eliminated, and a fresh slot is made in its place. The meniscus is prepared to a meniscal slot 1 cm in depth and 8 mm in width, and the slot is hand-prepared using rasps and a motorized burr. The remainder of the procedure is the same for primary meniscal transplantation with a bridge-in-slot technique.

Revision meniscal transplantation is rare; therefore, reports of outcomes are lacking. In the carefully selected young patient, however, it offers an option to improve knee function and decrease pain. Careful attention must be given to the identification of progressive articular cartilage disease, which should be treated concurrently with revision transplantation.

Strategies to Minimize Complications

The outcomes of meniscal transplantation are generally very good, with most studies reporting success rates near 85%.[10,11,20-22] Several clinical series have demonstrated decreased pain and improvement in range of motion. The most frequent complications after meniscal transplantation have been progressive articular cartilage degeneration and meniscal allograft degeneration. Successful outcome following transplantation also can be compromised by meniscal extrusion and tears of the transplanted meniscus.

Meniscal complications and failures often can be prevented. Patient selection is important, as is addressing all other knee pathology that may compromise the outcome of the meniscal transplant. Failure of the meniscal transplant often can be prevented by addressing malalignment with corrective osteotomy, ligamentous instability with ligament reconstruction, and focal cartilage defects with cartilage restorative procedures. These additional procedures can be performed simultaneously or in a staged fashion.[7,20,23]

Grafts are compartment specific and size specific. They are templated radiographically as described by Pollard et al.[24] Inaccurate measurements or inadequate size-matching can compromise the integrity of the graft, but the tolerance for graft size mismatch is not yet known. Oversized grafts can lead to greater articular cartilage contact pressures, and undersized grafts result in increased forces across the meniscus.[25]

Several surgical techniques have been described for meniscal allograft transplantation,[6-8] but we prefer a bridge-in-slot technique for both medial and lateral transplants. The advantages of the bone bridge technique are secure bony fixation, the ability to easily

© 2011 American Academy of Orthopaedic Surgeons

perform concomitant procedures, and the ability to maintain the native anterior and posterior meniscal horn attachments. Improper placement of anterior and posterior horn fixation sites may adversely affect the biomechanical function of the meniscus. The surgical technique becomes more complicated when concomitant procedures are performed, especially medial meniscal transplantation with ACL reconstruction, which has the added challenge of creating ACL tunnels and a meniscal slot that do not compromise either graft. Intraoperative complications such as bone block breakage and inadequate interference screw fixation can add to the complexity of the surgery. Familiarity with these complications and their treatment options are important to maximize outcomes and minimize stress levels in the operating room.

References

1. Voloshin AS, Wosk J: Shock absorption of meniscectomized and painful knees: A comparative in vivo study. *J Biomed Eng* 1983;5(2):157-161.
2. Walker PS, Erkman MJ: The role of the menisci in force transmission across the knee. *Clin Orthop Relat Res* 1975(109):184-192.
3. Levy IM, Torzilli PA, Warren RF: The effect of medial meniscectomy on anterior-posterior motion of the knee. *J Bone Joint Surg Am* 1982;64(6):883-888.
4. MacConaill MA: The movements of bones and joints: The synovial fluid and its assistants. *J Bone Joint Surg Br* 1950;32-B(2):244-252.
5. Renström P, Johnson RJ: Anatomy and biomechanics of the menisci. *Clin Sports Med* 1990;9(3):523-538.
6. Carter TR: Allograft meniscus transplantation: Dovetail technique, in Cole BJ, Sekiya JK, eds: *Surgical Techniques of the Shoulder, Elbow, and Knee in Sports Medicine.* Philadelphia, PA, Elsevier, 2008, pp 471-480.
7. Gomoll A, Farr J, Cole BJ: Allograft meniscus transplantation: Bridge in slot technique, in Cole BJ, Sekiya JK, eds: *Surgical Techniques of the Shoulder, Elbow, and Knee in Sports Medicine.* Philadelphia, PA, Elsevier, 2008, pp 459-470.
8. Jackson KR, Wickiewicz TL: Arthroscopic meniscus transplantation: Bone plug, in Cole BJ, Sekiya JK, eds: *Surgical Techniques of the Shoulder, Elbow, and Knee in Sports Medicine.* Philadelphia, PA, Elsevier, 2008, pp 481-490.
9. Bhosale AM, Myint P, Roberts S, et al: Combined autologous chondrocyte implantation and allogenic meniscus transplantation: A biological knee replacement. *Knee* 2007;14(5):361-368.
10. Farr J, Rawal A, Marberry KM: Concomitant meniscal allograft transplantation and autologous chondrocyte implantation: Minimum 2-year follow-up. *Am J Sports Med* 2007;35(9):1459-1466.
11. Rue JP, Yanke AB, Busam ML, McNickle AG, Cole BJ: Prospective evaluation of concurrent meniscus transplantation and articular cartilage repair: Minimum 2-year follow-up. *Am J Sports Med* 2008;36(9):1770-1778.
12. Gomoll AH, Kang RW, Chen AL, Cole BJ: Triad of cartilage restoration for unicompartmental arthritis treatment in young patients: Meniscus allograft transplantation, cartilage repair and osteotomy. *J Knee Surg* 2009;22(2):137-141.
13. Noyes FR, Mayfield W, Barber-Westin SD, Albright JC, Heckmann TP: Opening wedge high tibial osteotomy: An operative technique and rehabilitation program to decrease complications and promote early union and function. *Am J Sports Med* 2006;34(8):1262-1273.
14. Freedman KB, Nho SJ, Cole BJ: Marrow stimulating technique to augment meniscus repair. *Arthroscopy* 2003;19(7):794-798.
15. Adams JG, McAlindon T, Dimasi M, Carey J, Eustace S: Contribution of meniscal extrusion and cartilage loss to joint space narrowing in osteoarthritis. *Clin Radiol* 1999;54(8):502-506.
16. Gale DR, Chaisson CE, Totterman SM, Schwartz RK, Gale ME, Felson D: Meniscal subluxation: Association with osteoarthritis and joint space narrowing. *Osteoarthritis Cartilage* 1999;7(6):526-532.
17. Potter HG, Rodeo SA, Wickiewicz TL, Warren RF: MR imaging of meniscal allografts: Correlation with clinical and arthroscopic outcomes. *Radiology* 1996;198(2):509-514.
18. Verdonk PC, Verstraete KL, Almqvist KF, et al: Meniscal allograft transplantation: Long-term clinical results with radiological and magnetic resonance imaging correlations. *Knee Surg Sports Traumatol Arthrosc* 2006;14(8):694-706.
19. Roach CJ, Owens BD, DeBerardino TM: Revision of failed lateral meniscal allograft transplant. *Techn Knee Surg* 2009;8(1):64-66.
20. Cole BJ, Dennis MG, Lee SJ, et al: Prospective evaluation of allograft meniscus transplantation: A minimum 2-year follow-up. *Am J Sports Med* 2006;34(6):919-927.

© 2011 American Academy of Orthopaedic Surgeons

21. Sekiya JK, West RV, Groff YJ, Irrgang JJ, Fu FH, Harner CD: Clinical outcomes following isolated lateral meniscal allograft transplantation. *Arthroscopy* 2006;22(7): 771-780.
22. Verdonk PC, Demurie A, Almqvist KF, Veys EM, Verbruggen G, Verdonk R: Transplantation of viable meniscal allograft: Survivorship analysis and clinical outcome of one hundred cases. *J Bone Joint Surg Am* 2005;87(4):715-724.
23. Packer JD, Rodeo SA: Meniscal allograft transplantation. *Clin Sports Med* 2009;28(2):259-283, viii.
24. Pollard ME, Kang Q, Berg EE: Radiographic sizing for meniscal transplantation. *Arthroscopy* 1995;11(6): 684-687.
25. Dienst M, Greis PE, Ellis BJ, Bachus KN, Burks RT: Effect of lateral meniscal allograft sizing on contact mechanics of the lateral tibial plateau: An experimental study in human cadaveric knee joints. *Am J Sports Med* 2007;35(1):34-42.

© 2011 *American Academy of Orthopaedic Surgeons*

Chapter 7

Patellofemoral Cartilage Restoration and Tibial Tuberosity Osteotomies

Jack Farr II, MD

Introduction

Although patellofemoral cartilage is restored in the same technical manner as tibiofemoral cartilage, certain features are unique to the patellofemoral compartment. The patellofemoral compartment has unique biomechanical, kinematic, stability, and rehabilitation requirements. Most patellofemoral pain will respond to expert physical therapy with emphasis on a "core-to-the-floor" approach. Failure to adequately exhaust nonsurgical treatment is inexcusable. Besides the societal cost burden of unnecessary surgery, the debilitation of surgery may result in a knee that is in worse condition after surgery than before. For a patient whose condition fails to respond to a truly comprehensive therapy program, each pathoanatomic component of the patellofemoral problem must be defined in detail. This list should include the limb mechanical axis, rotation of the femur and tibia, status of medial and lateral soft tissues, patellar height, tibial tuberosity position, and regional mapping/grading of all articular cartilage lesions of the knee. This comprehensive list is used to formulate a plan of treatment to address each pathology. Historically, some clinicians espoused using a "proximal" or a "distal" surgery. Orthopaedic surgeons now appreciate the complexity of the patellofemoral compartment and realize that no Holy Grail exists; rather, each specific pathology requires appropriate specific treatment. The "proximal" and "distal" surgical schools of thought therefore must be merged. For example, in some cases a component of distal realignment/unloading will be needed to optimize proximal lateral and medial soft-tissue balancing, with the goal of normalizing the patellofemoral contact area, force, and stability. Even a technically correct "isolated" surgery that does not address each patellofemoral compartment pathology will fail to opti-

---

Dr. Farr or an immediate family member has received royalties from DePuy, Mitek, and Stryker; is a member of a speakers' bureau or has made paid presentations on behalf of DePuy and Genzyme; serves as a paid consultant to or is an employee of DePuy, Genzyme, Mitek, Zimmer, VOT, Advanced Biosurfaces, Tigenix, and Arthrex; has received research or institutional support from DePuy, Eli Lilly, Genzyme, Mitek, Regeneration Technologies, Smith & Nephew, Zimmer, Advanced Biosurfaces, and Osiris; and owns stock or stock options in Advanced Biosurfaces and VOT.

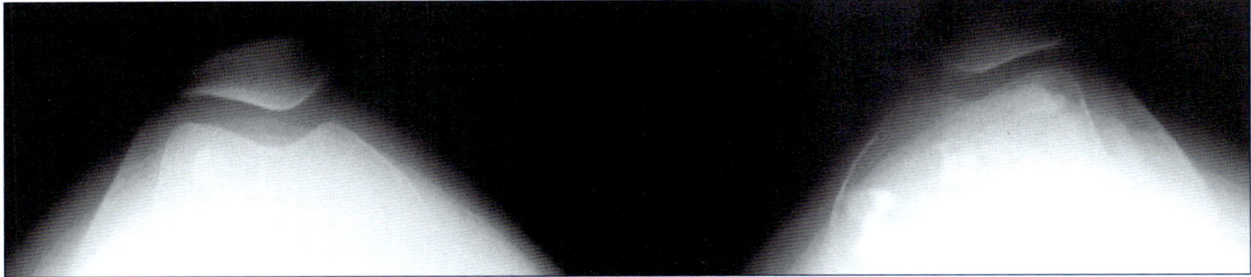

Figure 1 Merchant view of a patient with failed patellar autologous chondrocyte implantation in the left knee. Note that joint space is maintained.

mize the patient's comfort and function. Additionally, even with a correct diagnosis and proper surgical treatment, an improper postoperative rehabilitation program may not only result in a suboptimal outcome but can actually lead to failure if the cartilage restoration is subjected to inappropriate loading. As a result of the expected debilitation that occurs even with appropriate surgery, the patellofemoral compartment is very unforgiving. Multiple surgeries will increase the potential for complications as a result of scar formation and chronic muscular wasting.

Case 1: Delamination of Patellar Articular Cartilage

History

An 18-year-old woman with chronic static patellar subluxation (chronic excessive lateral patellar position relative to the trochlea) also had bipolar patellofemoral chondral lesions and a greater than normal tibial tuberosity–to–trochlear groove (TT-TG) distance (**Figure 1**). She was treated with bipolar autologous chondrocyte implantation (ACI), which is an off-label use in the United States, and anteromedialization (AMZ) osteotomy of the tibial tuberosity. The patient remained symptomatic after surgery. MRI and arthroscopy revealed delamination of the implanted patellar cartilage, marginal chondrosis progression at the patella, and integration of 50% of the trochlear implant. The TT-TG distance had been normalized, and the tilt was reversible. The patient underwent revision ACI with more aggressive marginal chondrosis débridement. After this revision treatment, the patient had progressive improvement in comfort, range of motion, and strength. Specific therapy was ordered to avoid overloading the patellofemoral compartment (ie, avoiding squats and concentrating on proximal core strengthening).

Current Problem

During the rehabilitation period, at 6 months after the surgery, the physical therapist independently decided the patient was making excellent progress and began a plyometric program of squats and box jumping, during which the patient experienced a pop and immediate pain and effusion. MRI revealed delamination of the revision patellar cartilage restoration (**Figure 2**).

Treatment

The patient underwent repeat débridement and staging for salvage cartilage restoration followed by appropriate rehabilitation.

Outcome

At 6 months after the repeat débridement, the patient was progressing well in therapy and reported improvement in her symptoms.

Discussion

Postoperative management is extremely important with all types of cartilage restoration. The pioneering work of Salter et al[1] showed that the cartilage healing process is sensitive to loading and motion. If too little motion or stress occurs, the cells may not be influenced toward a chondrocyte phenotype and thus may not participate actively to produce appropriate

© 2011 *American Academy of Orthopaedic Surgeons*

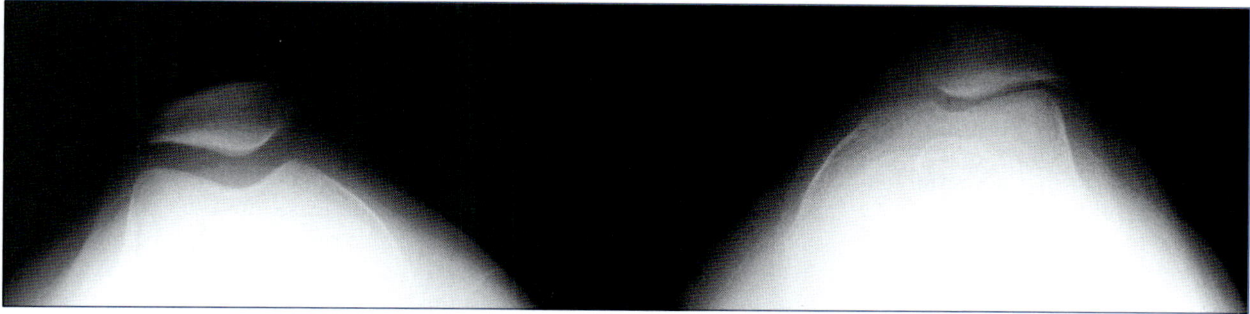

Figure 2 Merchant view of the same patient in Figure 1 shows left patellofemoral compartment narrowing after delamination of the patellar cartilage revision secondary to inappropriate rehabilitation.

hyaline-like matrix and aid in remodeling collagen in an optimal orientation to resist both shear and compressive loads. If the load is too great, the cells may be injured or the macroscopic structure may be disrupted. Overload may even lead to gross failure. Each type of cartilage restoration has a specific timeline for application of motion and stress that has been developed empirically by each technique's proponent. Until evidence-based medicine proves otherwise, a common-sense approach would be to follow the expert (level V evidence) guidelines for rehabilitation following the various cartilage restoration procedures.

Marrow Stimulation

Rehabilitation following marrow stimulation entails 6 to 8 weeks of non–weight bearing with either 8 hours per day of continuous passive motion or 500 unloaded cycles of knee flexion/extension three times per day, with gradual progression to full weight bearing as comfort and strength allow after that time. Return to previous activity levels may be possible at approximately 6 months.

Osteochondral Autograft Transplantation

Following an osteochondral autograft transplantation, crutch-assisted weight-bearing protection may be necessary for 2 to 6 weeks, depending on the number of plugs, the stability of the plugs, and the ability of the lesion shoulders to protect the plugs. The cartilage cap is mature, so "normal" cartilage is present and healing of the bone portion of the plug is complete at approximately 6 weeks; after that time, activities are progressed as motion, strength, and agility allow.

Osteochondral Allograft Transplantation

With an osteochondral allograft transplantation procedure, the cartilage is intact and ready for weight bearing, but the bone is dead and first must become incorporated at the base through initial bone-to-bone healing and then gradually through creeping substitution. Thus, the newer recommendations are to use as thin a shell of bone as possible. Because creeping substitution is a component of this procedure, the return to full activity is delayed compared with autograft but typically is earlier than with cell therapy. The exact timing depends on the size of the allograft, its position, and the thickness of the construct.

Chondrocyte Cell Therapy

Chondrocyte cell therapy in the United States uses cells in suspension; however, outside the United States, the options include suspension, suspension applied to a scaffold, and chondrocyte cells grown directly on a scaffold. The latter techniques may allow a jump start for the cells to begin producing matrix, but the process of maturation from immature, disorganized matrix to more mature matrix and then remodeled matrix still remains. The suggested schedule for early range of motion and loading is influenced by the specific type of implant, its size,

© 2011 American Academy of Orthopaedic Surgeons

and its position. The process may be somewhat slower in the patellofemoral compartment in light of the greater thickness of the patellar and trochlear cartilage compared with that of the tibiofemoral compartment. With the classic suspension cell therapies, the time to maximal potential loading may be as long as 18 to 24 months.

Preventing the Problem

Each cartilage restoration technique not only requires a unique rehabilitation approach for that technique but also has knee compartment–specific considerations. For example, patellofemoral cartilage restoration patients without other factors or surgeries may be allowed earlier full weight bearing with the knee braced straight, but they are restricted from stairs and inclines much longer than are patients who undergo similar cartilage techniques in the tibiofemoral compartment. Physical therapy (both patient-only and physical therapist–directed) plays a key role in the maturation process of the cartilage restoration. All team members (patient, surgeon, and therapist) must know the limitations and goals at each step of the process. Failure to adhere to the therapy program may be as devastating as failure at a biologic level.

Case 2: Complex Regional Pain Syndrome

History

A 34-year-old woman presented to her surgeon with activity-related patellofemoral pain and recurrent lateral instability. Nonsurgical measures failed to alleviate her symptoms. Plain radiographs were unremarkable. Arthroscopy and open lateral release were performed, followed by rehabilitation, but the patient reported increased instability and increased constant, burning pain.

Current Problem

Examination revealed pain disproportionate to the objective examination of the limb, which is classic for complex regional pain syndrome. Range of motion was full. There was marked quadriceps debilitation. Both medial and lateral patellar displacement elicited further increase in pain and apprehension.

Treatment

The patient underwent a series of paralumbar sympathetic blocks and pain management until the pain was primarily activity-related. MRI revealed extensive medial patellar chondrosis, redundancy of the medial patellofemoral ligament (MPFL), and an extensive prior lateral release into the vastus lateralis. The Caton-Deschamps ratio was normal, and the TT-TG distance was 22 mm (**Figure 3**). The patient underwent an extensive proximal core rehabilitation program. Staging arthroscopy confirmed the presence of intra-articular patellar chondral pathology, and plans were made for salvage surgery.

The patient underwent reconstruction of the medial and lateral patellofemoral ligaments concomitant with cartilage restoration of the patella and AMZ to normalize the TT-TG distance (**Figure 4**). The surgery was performed under regional blocks as well as a paralumbar sympathetic block in an attempt to minimize the reactivation of sympathetically mediated pain.

Outcome

The patient was followed closely by an expert patellofemoral therapist and a pain management specialist and gradually experienced resolution of disabling knee pain. The medial and lateral patellar instability resolved completely.

Discussion

Most patellofemoral surgeries affect the stress to the patellofemoral articular cartilage, so it is important to consider the positive and negative factors with all patellofemoral surgeries. Rehabilitation and pain management are crucial for optimizing any surgical outcome.

Lateral release is not a panacea. In fact, despite the common use of lateral release, the indications for it have become progressively more limited and focused over the past 10 years, as evidenced by a 2008 poll of the International Patellofemoral Study Group (unpublished data). Surgeons in the group who performed a high volume of patellofemoral surgeries performed lateral releases in less than 2% of their cases. Lateral release may be easy to perform, but complications are not unusual and can include hemarthrosis or hematoma requiring surgery, chronic quadriceps weakness, increased lateral instability

© 2011 American Academy of Orthopaedic Surgeons

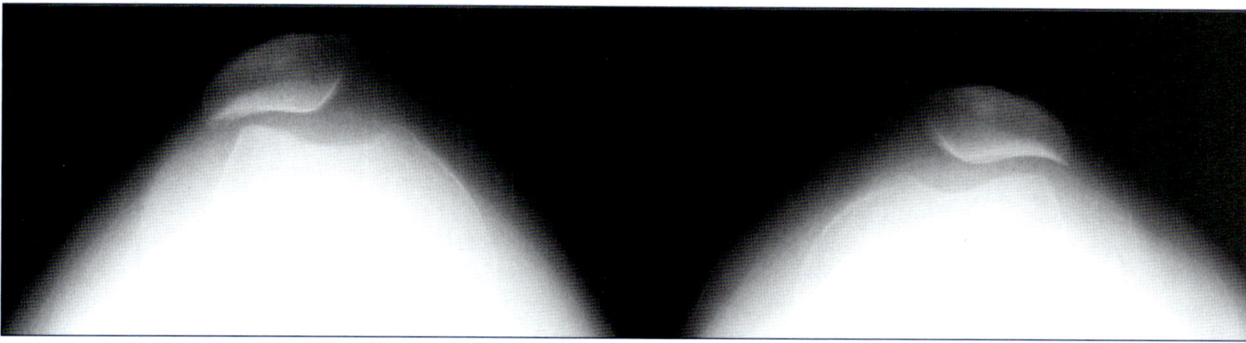

Figure 3 Preoperative Merchant view shows maintenance of the joint space and mild centrolateral position of the patella in the left knee. An MRI (not shown) separately demonstrated a greater than normal tibial tubercle–to–trochlear groove (TT-TG) distance.

Figure 4 Merchant view of the same patient in Figure 3 after anteromedialization (AMZ), shows a central patella in the left knee. Stäubli et al[7] demonstrated that the bone contours do not always follow the cartilage contours, so mild apparent subluxation may be present, even after surgery.

(the lateral retinaculum does participate in limiting lateral patellar displacement), iatrogenic medial patellar instability, and complex regional pain syndrome.

The MPFL is the "essential," or primary, restraint to pathologic lateral patellar displacement. Clinical studies with level I evidence show no statistical superiority of MPFL repair over nonsurgical management.[2,3] On the other hand, MPFL reconstruction series demonstrate very low rates of recurrence with some level III and IV evidence. Level IV evidence MPFL repair series show promise with some types of repair, but high levels of evidence-based medicine are needed. With both MPFL repair and reconstruction, advocates agree that it is important to identify the MPFL pathology and correct it anatomically rather than globally reefing or advancing medial structures.

Recognizing the Problem

Complex regional pain syndrome and subset (sympathetically mediated pain) variants are not uncommon with any knee injury or surgery. Early recognition is the key to resolution, and an early, specific sympathetic block is essential to the diagnosis. A sympathetic block is also the first part of the multimodal treatment, which involves oral agents, comprehensive physical therapy, and appropriate loading exercises.

Preventing the Problem

The first step in preventing the problem is to thoroughly analyze the patient presentation and the status of the limb. After that, focus should shift to the knee, and finally to the patellofemoral joint and its cartilage. The patellofemoral compartment has unique characteristics. Fortunately, increasing levels

© 2011 American Academy of Orthopaedic Surgeons

of objective data are becoming available on the role of medial and lateral soft tissues and options for tibial tuberosity osteotomy. Some of the newer concepts have not been published in textbooks, but they are described in "current concept" reviews in peer-reviewed journals and in monographs. Although the patellofemoral surgical techniques may vary minimally from those described more than 20 years ago, the algorithms for specific applications have changed. In addition to a thorough history and physical examination and plain radiography, current MRI evaluation can yield information on the status of the MPFL and injury site, the patellar height (Caton-Deschamps ratio), TT-TG distance, bone bruising, and sites of chondral or osteochondral injuries.

Case 3: Postoperative Fracture

History

A 32-year-old woman presented with chronic anterolateral knee pain. Clinically, the Q angle appeared to be within normal limits. After failed nonsurgical management, a contained chondral lesion of the lateral trochlea was noted on MRI and confirmed as the only intra-articular pathology. The lesion was treated with microfracture. Empirically, a lateral release was performed to unload the lateral lesion. No postoperative complications occurred.

Current Problem

Strength recovery was slow but was gradually achieved. After strength recovery, the patient continued to have pain proportionate to activity, especially with patellofemoral loading, similar to that experienced preoperatively. Radiographs showed full joint space maintenance, normal patellar height, and a central patella.

Treatment

MRI demonstrated repair fill and mild subchondral bone edema at the site of the microfracture, and a greater than normal TT-TG distance. The patient underwent AMZ to unload the region of cartilage restoration. She was then treated with aggressive rehabilitation. She was weaned from crutches at 3 weeks. Upon making a twisting motion, she noted a pop in her tibia. Radiographs demonstrated a nondisplaced fracture at the site of the AMZ (**Figure 5**). The patient was treated with casting, and the fracture healed uneventfully. Upon completion of therapy, the patient was pain free.

Discussion

Recognizing the Problem

Stress risers are created with any bone intervention, and they predispose the bone to fracture at lower levels of energy than in the preoperative state. In patellofemoral interventions, the two areas of most concern are the patella after drilling tunnels for MPFL reconstruction and the tibia after AMZ (more so than straight medialization). Strict adherence to weight-bearing restrictions has decreased the incidence of fracture after AMZ. Delayed patellar fractures have been reported after drilling patellar tunnels for MPFL reconstruction. Such fractures may be avoided by using techniques that do not require tunnels.[4]

Preventing the Problem

Cartilage restoration is rarely performed in isolation. The patellofemoral compartment is subjected to very high loads, even with activities of daily living (eg, loading with stair climbing is equal to several times body weight). AMZ is a common unloading procedure used with cartilage restoration but is much more structurally invasive than a straight medialization (Elmslie-Trillat procedure). After a report was published on fractures with accelerated weight bearing after AMZ, 6 weeks of minimal weight bearing has been recommended.[5] Straight medialization would rarely play a role in conjunction with cartilage restoration, as the goal is to decrease the load to the restored tissue. Therefore, AMZ is more commonly applied when the tuberosity is excessively lateral and patellar cartilage is restored.

The loading of planned regions of restoration must be considered. The environment should be evaluated with MRI to document contact areas, subchondral edema, and the measurements of tuberosity position and patellar height. The patellofemoral loads are optimized before or concomitant with patellofemoral cartilage restoration. Strict adherence to rehabilitation guidelines is essential to success.

 © 2011 American Academy of Orthopaedic Surgeons

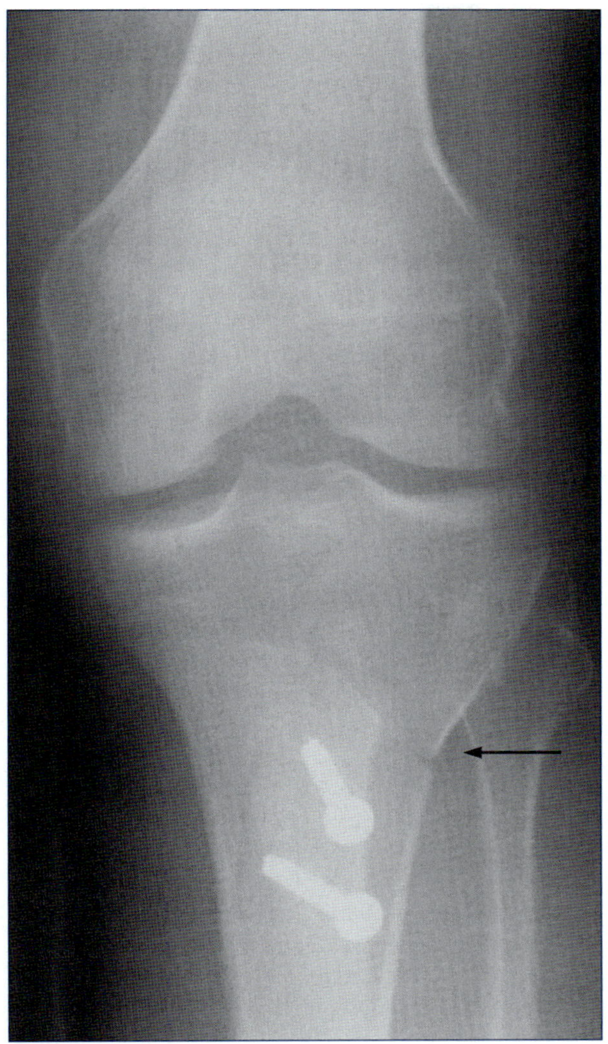

Figure 5 AP radiograph shows a nondisplaced tibial fracture (arrow) at the level of the AMZ.

Additional Strategies to Minimize the Risk of Complications

Neurovascular Complications

The popliteal and anterior tibial arteries are near the surgical field of tibial tuberosity procedures. Screw fixation can compromise either artery, and with AMZ, both the anterior tibial artery and deep peroneal nerve are at risk of injury if not properly protected (**Figure 6**). With MPFL reconstruction and repair, the saphenous nerve or, more frequently, one of the infrapatellar branches of the saphenous nerve may be injured. Both of these nerves are associated with complex regional (sympathetically mediated) pain syndrome, which requires early and aggressive management. In addition, any incision about the knee can lead to small but highly symptomatic neuromas that cannot be ignored.[6]

Compartment Syndrome

With the anterior compartment elevation from the lateral wall of the tibia and subsequent retractor pressure during an AMZ, compartment syndrome is a risk. Loose reapproximation at closure and meticulous hemostasis are instrumental in decreasing the possibility of compartment syndrome. When compartment syndrome does occur, early recognition and management are key in optimizing the final outcome.

Arthrofibrosis and Patella Infera

Arthrofibrosis and patella infera can occur with any surgery or trauma. Arthrofibrosis is a multifactorial process—probably with an underlying biologic predisposition. Nevertheless, potential triggering factors can be minimized by taking extra measures to achieve meticulous hemostasis and minimize early swelling, by prescribing early range of motion as allowed by the procedures, and by recognizing and treating atypical pain.

Failure to Recognize Femoral and/or Tibial Torsional Abnormalities

Many cases of malalignment can be traced to the tibial tuberosity, but it is not the only source. Some patients have rotational (axial plane) or tibiofemoral (coronal plane) malalignment. Although it seems obvious to point out that malalignment should be treated at the source (eg, distal femoral varus osteotomy for valgus malalignment and external derotational osteotomy for excessive femoral anteversion), it is important to have a high level of suspicion during the physical examination for malalignment proximal and distal to the knee. For concerns

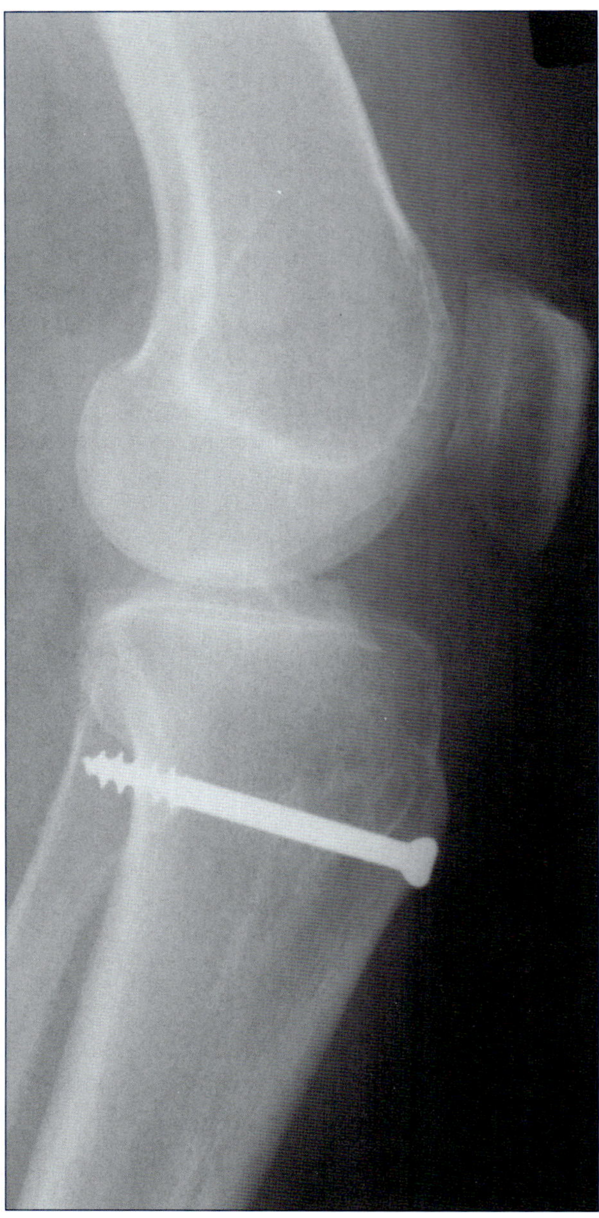

Figure 6 Lateral radiograph shows anterior-to-posterior direction of an excessively long screw that placed vascularity at risk. Screws should be directed posteromedially and be of proper length.

about tibiofemoral coronal plane malalignment, a hip-to-ankle weight-bearing radiograph will avoid mismanagement. For rotational assessment, a prone physical evaluation of internal and external rotation of the hips should be included. If abnormal rotation is suspected, a CT scan of the hip, knee, and ankle will allow delineation of rotational alignment.

Overzealous Surgery

The goal of patellofemoral surgery is to normalize/optimize stability, force transmission, and contact area. More of any specific surgery is certainly not better; for example, overmedialization increases not only medial patellofemoral force but also medial tibiofemoral force; excessive lateral release may not only create medial instability but also may decrease restraint to lateral displacement forces; and excessive medial shortening or malpositioning of an MPFL attachment site will overload the medial patellofemoral compartment, with expected consequences. Emphasis on normalization/optimization will decrease these avoidable complications.

Summary

A rehabilitation program should be exhausted before proceeding with surgical planning. Surgery, when indicated, is based on normalizing each component of the pathology involving the limb, the knee, and the patellofemoral compartment. In the patellofemoral compartment, it is clear that no single surgical solution exists. Surgical intervention depends on the pathoanatomy and may include proximal medial, proximal lateral, and tuberosity surgery, as well as cartilage restoration. Each type of surgical intervention carries an inherent risk that can be minimized by respecting anatomy and closely adhering to established surgical techniques. After a well-planned and well-executed surgery, the patient and physical therapist must follow the prescribed rehabilitation protocol closely.

© 2011 *American Academy of Orthopaedic Surgeons*

References

1. Salter RB, Simmonds DF, Malcolm BW, Rumble EJ, MacMichael D, Clements ND: The biological effect of continuous passive motion on the healing of full-thickness defects in articular cartilage: An experimental investigation in the rabbit. *J Bone Joint Surg Am* 1980;62(8):1232-1251.
2. Christiansen SE, Jakobsen BW, Lund B, Lind M: Isolated repair of the medial patellofemoral ligament in primary dislocation of the patella: A prospective randomized study. *Arthroscopy* 2008;24(8):881-887.
3. Nikku R, Nietosvaara Y, Aaleo K, Kallio PE: Operative treatment of primary patellar dislocation does not improve medium-term outcome: A 7-year follow-up report and risk analysis of 127 randomized patients. *Acta Orthop* 2005;76(5):699-704.
4. Thaunat M, Erasmus PJ: Recurrent patellar dislocation after medial patellofemoral ligament reconstruction. *Knee Surg Sports Traumatol Arthrosc* 2008;16(1): 40-43.
5. Stetson WB, Friedman MJ, Fulkerson JP, Cheng M, Buuck D: Fracture of the proximal tibia with immediate weightbearing after a Fulkerson osteotomy. *Am J Sports Med* 1997;25(4):570-574.
6. Fulkerson JP, Tennant R, Jaivin JS, Grunnet M: Histologic evidence of retinacular nerve injury associated with patellofemoral malalignment. *Clin Orthop Relat Res* 1985(197):196-205.
7. Stäubli HU, Dürrenmatt U, Porcellini B, Rauschning W: Anatomy and surface geometry of the patellofemoral joint in the axial plane. *J Bone Joint Surg Br* 1999;81(3):452-458.

© 2011 *American Academy of Orthopaedic Surgeons*

Index

*Page numbers followed by *f* indicate figures; page numbers followed by *t* indicate tables.

© 2011 *American Academy of Orthopaedic Surgeons*

L

M

N

O

© 2011 *American Academy of Orthopaedic Surgeons*

P

R

S

T

V

© 2011 American Academy of Orthopaedic Surgeons